....

Amsterdam Growth and Health Longitudinal Study

Medicine and Sport Science

Vol. 47

Series Editors

J. Borms   *Brussels*
M. Hebbelinck   *Brussels*
A.P. Hills   *Brisbane*

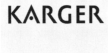

....

Amsterdam Growth and Health Longitudinal Study (AGAHLS)

A 23-Year Follow-Up from Teenager to Adult about Lifestyle and Health

Volume Editor

H.C.G. Kemper   *Amsterdam*

50 figures, 3 in color, and 39 tables, 2004

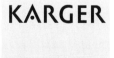

Basel · Freiburg · Paris · London · New York ·
Bangalore · Bangkok · Singapore · Tokyo · Sydney

Medicine and Sport Science

Founder and Editor from 1969 to 1984: E. Jokl[†], Lexington, Ky.

·····················

Prof. Dr. Han C.G. Kemper

AGAHLS Research Group
EMGO Institute
VU University Medical Center
Van der Boechorststraat 7
NL–1081 BT Amsterdam
The Netherlands
hcg.kemper.emgo@med.vu.nl

Library of Congress Cataloging-in-Publication Data

Amsterdam growth and health longitudinal study (AGAHLS) : a 23-year follow-up from
    teenager to adult about lifestyle and health / volume editor,
    H.C.G. Kemper.
        p. ; cm. – (Medicine and sport science, ISSN 0254–5020 ; v. 47)
    Includes bibliographical references and index.
    ISBN 3–8055–7652–8 (hard cover : alk. paper)
        1. Health behavior–Netherlands–Amsterdam–Longitudinal studies.   2. Health
    attitudes–Netherlands–Amsterdam–Longitudinal studies.   3. Lifestyles–Health
    aspects–Netherlands–Amsterdam–Longitudinal studies.   4. Youth–Health and
    hygiene–Netherlands–Amsterdam–Longitudinal studies.   5. Young adults–Health and
    hygiene–Netherlands–Amsterdam–Longitudinal studies.   I. Kemper, Han C. G. II. Series,
    [DNLM: 1. Health Behavior–Adolescent–Netherlands.   2. Health
    Behavior–Adult–Netherlands.   3. Life Style–Adolescent–Netherlands.   4. Life
    Style–Adult–Netherlands.   5. Longitudinal Studies–Netherlands.   6. Risk
    Factors–Adolescent–Netherlands.   7. Risk Factors–Adult–Netherlands.   8. Risk Reduction
    Behavior–Adolescent–Netherlands.   9. Risk Reduction Behavior–Adult–Netherlands. W
    85 A528 2004]
    RA776.9.A478 2004
    613'.09492'352–dc22

                                                                    2003063487

Bibliographic Indices. This publication is listed in bibliographic services, including Current Contents® and Index Medicus.

Drug Dosage. The authors and the publisher have exerted every effort to ensure that drug selection and dosage set forth in this text are in accord with current recommendations and practice at the time of publication. However, in view of ongoing research, changes in government regulations, and the constant flow of information relating to drug therapy and drug reactions, the reader is urged to check the package insert for each drug for any change in indications and dosage and for added warnings and precautions. This is particularly important when the recommended agent is a new and/or infrequently employed drug.

© Copyright 2004 by S. Karger AG, P.O. Box, CH–4009 Basel (Switzerland)
www.karger.com
Printed in Switzerland on acid-free paper by Reinhardt Druck, Basel
ISSN 0254–5020
ISBN 3–8055–7652–8

....

Contents

....
Preface

This third monograph of the Amsterdam Growth and Health Longitudinal Study (AGAHLS) reports on trends in life-style and health from the ages of 13 to 36. Longitudinal studies with a follow-up lasting for a quarter of a century are very rare, and the AGAHLS is unique among them for several reasons. Firstly, the focus is truly multidisciplinary and involves both physical and psychological determinants in relation to a wide range of health outcomes. Secondly, the multiple measurements were carefully standardized in nine waves of data collection, thus producing a high-quality data set. Thirdly, the AGAHLS has had a surprisingly low rate of loss to follow-up and has succeeded in the prevention of bias due to its sophisticated design. Fourthly, the longitudinal data have been analyzed very efficiently by the application of advanced statistical techniques.

This monograph not only provides an overview of 23 years of follow-up, but it also elegantly summarizes over 200 scientific publications and 10 PhD theses. The AGAHLS is a cohort study in many ways. The core cohort was, of course, originally formed by the 12- and 13-year-old participants from two Dutch secondary schools. For them, the study has become a regular event in their lives, and has provided an opportunity to keep in touch with their former classmates. Their partners and children were also invited to attend the reunion in 2001, and this identified two related cohorts. Yet another cohort consists of all the dedicated workers and students who made the AGAHLS such a scientific success by their contribution to the data collection. A very special sub-cohort in this respect is formed by the PhD students, of which a subgroup already became assistant or associate professor.

Although the AGAHLS is very much a group product, there is one central person who forms the driving force and is the single most important determinant of its success. Han Kemper had the vision, the ambition and the stamina, all of which are essential in longitudinal research. In addition to being a scientist who has gained substantial international esteem, including two honorary doctorates, he is also an extremely nice person and a champion in motivation, inspiration and fund-raising. This monograph marks his retirement from Academia, and it therefore seems appropriate to dedicate this volume to its Editor.

Lex M. Bouter, Amsterdam

Kemper HCG (ed): Amsterdam Growth and Health Longitudinal Study.
Med Sport Sci. Basel, Karger, 2004, vol 47, pp 1–4

....

Genesis of the Study and Acknowledgements to Subjects, Authors, Researchers and Sponsors

Han C.G. Kemper

Institute for Research in Extramural Medicine (EMGO Institute),
VU University Medical Center (VUmc), Amsterdam, The Netherlands

'This volume in the series of *Medicine and Sport Sciences* is devoted to the research of growth, health and fitness of teenagers, the generation that will bring forth the top athletes of the eighties.' This was my first sentence in the preface of the first monograph of the Amsterdam Growth and Health Longitudinal Study, publishing the results of four annual measurements of teenage boys and girls in 1985 [1].

'The longitudinal data reported in this HK Sport Science Monograph are from a 15-year multidisciplinary study carried out in youngsters.' This was my first sentence in the preface of the second monograph of the Amsterdam Growth and Health Longitudinal Study, publishing the results of the same population covering the age span from 13 to 27 years with in total six repeated measurements in 1995 [2].

The present publication marks a period of almost a quarter of a century of follow-up of our subjects.

In this volume the authors show the strength of a carefully performed longitudinal study, aimed at a low drop out rate and standardized procedures of repeated measurements over the years.

The main objective of this third monograph is threefold: firstly to analyze the changes in health, fitness and lifestyles and secondly to calculate the relationships between changes in lifestyle and health in a healthy population of Dutch youngsters from age 13 till the adult age of 36 years.

Although the changes in lifestyles such as physical activity, eating, alcohol consumption and smoking are taken as determinants for health characteristics, the results from our descriptive study cannot be considered on the basis of cause and effect.

A third objective was to ascertain the stability and predictability of determinants (such as physical activity and dietary intake, smoking and alcohol consumption) on the outcomes (biological risk factors for cardiovascular diseases, osteoporosis and obesity).

During the study period we added important newly developed noninvasive techniques, such as dual X-ray absorptiometry (DEXA) to measure bone mineral mass, ultrasound of carotid and femoral arteries to measure atherosclerosis and stiffness and also determination of DNA in the blood to relate polymorphisms with risk factors for chronic diseases.

We were also able to evaluate the effects of health information by a natural experiment. In 1996, we included the subjects who served as controls during the teenage period at age 13–16 years for a second follow-up together with our longitudinal group. The differences at age 32 of both groups on biologic risk factors, physical activity and dietary intake are supposed to be the effects of health information during the 20-year follow-up period.

The Amsterdam Growth and Health Longitudinal study was inspired by the Nijmegen Growth Study [3] which followed Dutch children from age 4 to 14 years. The Tecumseh Community Health Study [4] was another world-famous study that was the first to include physical activity data in their collection of a whole population living in a natural community ranging from 10 to 69 years of age.

Recently, a monograph was published from the famous Seven Countries Study [5] which includes results about prevention of coronary heart disease (CHD) over a period of 40 years, including measurements of diet, lifestyle and CHD risk factors in a sample from Zutphen in the Netherlands.

Acknowledgements

First, I would like to acknowledge the members of the research team that collected all the data at the last measurement period (2000): Mrs Ir Ingrid Bakker, Mrs Eveline HCM Bekkering, Mrs Dr. Claire M Bernaards, Mrs Dr. Isabel Ferreira, Dr. Lando LJ Koppes, Dr. Jan Snel, Mrs Dr. Saskia J. te Velde, Mrs Wieke de Vente, and always in the background Mrs Ank Versteegh, Dr. Jos W.R. Twisk and Prof. Dr. Willem van Mechelen.

Students who undertook their research with this study included Mrs Ellen Althuizen, Mrs Sophia de Graaff, Leander Heyink, Yvonne de Jong and Ralph van Wijnckel. Mrs Sagita Soechitram, Mrs Thelma Vreden and Mrs Christy Niemeyer, MD, acted as research assistants.

Mrs Lisanne Warmerdam took care of all the collected data and managed the integration of the 2000 data into the longitudinal database. The AGAHLS

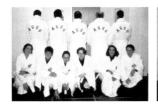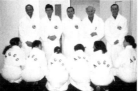

Fig. 1. The research group in 2000.

data base, with detailed description of the methods and value labels, is available for other researchers on request to perform secondary analyses in the NIWI / Steinmetz Archive (Amsterdam, The Netherlands).

Figure 1: The Research Group in 2000

As always it was a period during which we worked 6 days a week (including many Saturdays) in order to measure as many of our subjects as possible. A special tribute to Wieke de Vente who was the perfect and charming manager in organizing the daily schedule, reception of the subjects during most of the measurement days between February and June 2000.

We were able to maximize the adherence rate: 450 male and females were measured, about two thirds of the population of 600 we started with in 1976. Thousands of phone calls, e-mails, postmails and faxes were sent by our team to contact our subjects, to make appointments for a suitable day and to mail the necessary forms and disposables to prepare themselves on the measurement day.

All these men and women who gave their time and effort to share with us their physical and mental state of health and insights in their lifestyle, were invaluable in contributing to the success of this longitudinal study.

Principle Responsibility

This AGAHLS is carried out at the VU University Medical Center in the Institute for Research in Extramural Medicine (EMGO) in Amsterdam, The Netherlands. The Medical Ethical Committee of the Vrije Universiteit Amsterdam approved the protocol.

It is a research project within the program Prevention and Health Promotion of the Netherlands School of Primary Care Research (CaRe). CaRe was in 1995 acknowledged by the Royal Netherlands Academy of Arts and Sciences (KNAW).

Financial Support

The AGAHLS received financial support from the Netherlands Heart Foundation in The Hague (NHS), The Dutch Prevention Fund in The Hague (currently ZONmw), the Dutch Ministry of Well Being and Public Health in The Hague (VWS), the Dairy Foundation on Nutrition and Health in Zoetermeer (NZO), the Dutch Olympic Committee/the Netherlands Sports Federation in Arnhem (NOC*NSF), Heineken Inc. in Zoetermeer, and the Scientific Board of Smoking and Health in The Hague.

This Monograph

The publication of this third monograph is a milestone for AGAHLS. Although more than 200 international publications are published over the last 25 years about our study, a summary publication such as this in the Karger Series *Medicine and Sport Science* is an important and valuable source that can be used by researchers, teachers and students in the field of growth, aging, health, exercise, nutrition and longitudinal data.

The first monograph (1985) and the constituent articles therein were cited more than 100 times in the (social sciences) citation index.

My two secretaries Ank Versteegh and Sophal Varossieau were very helpful in preparing the draft for this.

We thank the series editors J. Borms, M. Hebbelinck and A.P. Hills for their willingness to accept this publication in their highly esteemed series and Karger publishers for their always professional editing and production.

References

1   Kemper HCG (ed): In Hebbelinck M (series ed): Growth, health and fitness of teenagers – Longitudinal research in international perspective. Med Sport Sci. Basel, Karger, 1985, vol 20.
2   Kemper HCG (ed): The Amsterdam Growth Study. A longitudinal analysis of health, fitness, and lifestyle. HK Sport Science Monograph Series. Champaign, Human Kinetics, 1995, vol 6.
3   Prahl-Andersen B, Kowalski CJ, Heydendael P: A Mixed Longitudinal Interdisciplinary Study of Growth and Development. New York, Academic Press, 1994.
4   Montoye HJ: Physical Activity and Health: An Epidemiological Study of an Entire Community. Englewood Cliffs, Prentice-Hall, 1975.
5   Kromhout D, Menotti A, Blackburn H: Prevention of Coronary Heart Disease – Diet, Lifestyle and Risk Factors in the Seven Countries Study. Dordrecht, Kluwer, 2002.

Han C.G. Kemper
Principle investigator of AGAHLS and editor of this volume.

Kemper HCG (ed): Amsterdam Growth and Health Longitudinal Study.
Med Sport Sci. Basel, Karger, 2004, vol 47, pp 5–20

....

General Introduction

Han C.G. Kemper[a], J. Snel[b], Willem van Mechelen[c]

[a] Institute for Research in Extramural Medicine (EMGO Institute),
   VU University Medical Center (VUmc),
[b] Department of Psychology, University of Amsterdam, and
[c] Institute for Research in Extramural Medicine and Department of Social Medicine,
   VU University Medical Center, Amsterdam, The Netherlands

Birth of the AGAHLS

In 1974, a longitudinal study was planned to monitor the growth, health and life-style, over a period of 4 years, of boys and girls entering secondary school. The reason for this follow-up was a series of intervention studies to measure the effectiveness of more intensive and extra physical education lessons in 12- to 13-year-old boys [1, 2]. In general, no clear effects were found. There were indications that large interindividual differences between the pupils in biological development and habitual physical activity could have masked any intervention effects. At that time, health authorities were complaining about the level of fitness of youngsters in their late teens. In growing towards independence, the life-style habits of teenager's change considerably (with regard to physical activity, food intake, and tobacco smoking and alcohol consumption). Thereby, their health perspective may also change. This illustrates that the teenage period is an important period in life. Individual changes in growth and development can be described most precisely by studying the same participants over a longer period of time. That is what led to the birth of the Amsterdam Growth and Health Longitudinal Study (AGAHLS).

The AGAHLS started by following a sample of over 600 healthy 13-year-old boys and girls with four annual measurements. The boys and girls were pupils from two secondary schools (one in Amsterdam and one in Purmerend, a suburb of Amsterdam). The follow-up was extended with measurements at the ages of 21, 27, 29 and 32 years. In 2000, almost 400 (36-year-old) participants

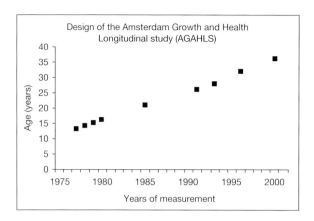

Fig. 1. Design of the Amsterdam Growth and Health Longitudinal Study. On the vertical axis age (in years) and on the horizontal axis the years of measurements.

attended the ninth measurement session, so that 23-year follow-up data are available now (fig. 1).

This longitudinal database covers the important teenage and (young) adult period, and makes it possible to analyze the data to determine the tracking characteristics of biological and life-style variables, and also to investigate quasi-causal relationships between life-style variables and indicators for some chronic diseases. Moreover, new techniques, such as the measurement of early signs of atherosclerosis and osteoporosis, and genetic markers for chronic diseases have been added to the database, and are related to the longitudinal data that have been collected previously from the same participants.

In 2001, a reunion was organized to celebrate the 25th anniversary of the AGAHLS. Because most of the participants are now in an age period that they have started a family and are bringing up children, their spouses and children were also invited (fig. 2). At this reunion, the participants received a popular Dutch version of the 1995 AGAHLS monograph [3], which was published for them and for other interested lay people [4].

Objectives

Initial Period: Growth, Health and Fitness of Teenagers (1974–1983)
In the 1970s, this longitudinal study was initially designed to answer the following four research questions:
1 How do boys and girls grow and develop with respect to their physical and social-psychological well-being between the ages of 12 and 18?

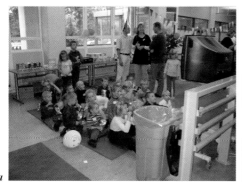
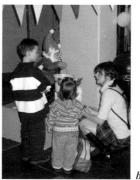
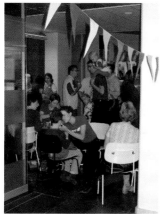

Fig. 2. Impression of the reunion on the occasion of the silver jubilee of the AGAHLS on October 6th, 2001.

2   How does the life-style change, particularly in those aspects that seem important for health?
3   How healthy are these teenagers, and how healthy is their life-style with respect to diet, physical activity, smoking behavior and alcohol consumption?
4   What relationship can be discovered between life-style and health?

In 1976, a 6-year grant was obtained from the Foundation for Educational Research (Dutch Ministry of Education) and the Dutch Prevention Fund (currently Health Research and Development Council [ZONmw]) for the initiation of this longitudinal study. In view of the many confounding factors, inevitably connected with longitudinal measurements, a multiple longitudinal study was designed, to enable confounding of 'time of measurement' and 'birth cohort' to be separated from the main 'age effect'. Therefore, in 1976, from a school in Amsterdam (Pius X) entire school classes were selected, with approximately 300 pupils from three different birth cohorts (1963, 1964 and 1965),

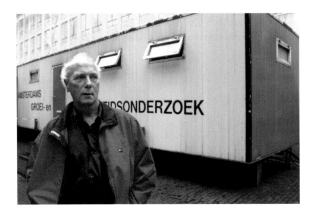

Fig. 3. Last picture of the 30-year-old mobile research laboratory on the VU campus.

and four annual repeated measurements (1977, 1978, 1979 and 1980) were carried out.

Another problem encountered in longitudinal measurements is a testing or learning effect. When measuring many variables – physical as well as psychological – a certain motivation or habituation is required from the participants. This can lead to differences between measurements that are solely due to changes in attitude towards the measurement procedure itself. Such testing effects may be positive (i.e. when habituation or learning is important), or negative (i.e. when motivation decreases). Therefore, a control group in which no repeated measurements were made was included in the AGAHLS: at a second school in Purmerend (Ignatius College). The same measurements were performed on approximately 300 pupils (comparable with those of the first school), but only once during the entire 4-year period, measuring only 25% of the pupils each year. The measurements of this 'control' school were comparable with those of the 'longitudinal' school, except that they were not repeated measurements, but were derived from independent samples [5]. Comparing the data from the two schools, possible systematic divergence of mean values over age is an indication of a testing effect. The multiple longitudinal design made it possible to estimate confounding effects that can interfere with the main age effects during the first four adolescent years, including drop-out effects and stochastic measurement errors [6].

The data-collection was facilitated by a mobile research lab that was transported by trailer from the longitudinal school to the control school, and vice versa. Thereafter the lab was placed at the VUmc. In 2002, after almost 30 years of excellent service, the mobile research lab was dismantled after a new lab was installed in the VUmc (fig. 3).

The results over the teenage period show clearly that, although physical fitness and health do not decline during this period in either boys or girls, habitual physical activity (measured by pedometers, heart rate monitors and interviews) declined dramatically. Further, eating habits were characterized by a constant pattern of an intake too high in fat and protein and too low in carbohydrate content. A significant increase was seen in the percentage of smokers and alcohol consumers [7].

Second Period: The Amsterdam Growth and Health Longitudinal Study (1983–1995)

The results over the initial period inferred continuation of this 4-year longitudinal study to find out whether a continuation or deterioration of these life-styles would ultimately be manifested in favorable physical and psychosocial characteristics in adulthood, and to find out what direction the changes would have taken at a young adult age. Grants from several organizations in the Netherlands (Dutch Heart Foundation, Health Research and Development Council, Ministry of Health, Welfare and Sport, Dairy Foundation on Nutrition and Health, NOC*NSF) enabled the study to be continued. The participants of the longitudinal study were measured again at the mean age of 21 years in 1985 and at the mean ages of 27 and 29 years in 1991 and 1993.

The measurement of a different age group demanded a critical update, so some new measurements were included and others were left out. Included were measurements of stress and isokinetic leg muscle force in 1985 and 1991. The bone density determinations of the lumbar region in 1991 and of the hip and wrist in 1993. The DEXA measurements were done with cooperation with the Department of Nuclear Medicine (Prof. J. Teule, Dr. J.C. Roos and Dr. P.T.A.M. Lips) of the VUmc. The assessment of skeletal age was left out, because full maturity was reached in all participants.

Results over this 15-year follow-up period show an increase in a series of risk indicators for cardiovascular diseases (CVD). For example, at the age of 27, one third of the population was overweight (Body Mass Index ≥ 25), but also blood pressure and cholesterol levels had increased considerably [8]. These findings indicate that even at the age of 27 (and probably before), preventive strategies to reduce fat mass and the serum cholesterol profile may be of great importance.

One important aspect of the AGAHLS was the repeated measurement of various aspects of life-style, including nutritional intake, physical activity, and behavioral patterns such as stress and coping style. The descriptive nature of the AGAHLS does not justify the drawing of firm conclusions about the effects of life-style and psychosocial patterns on health. However, modern statistical methods, such as longitudinal analysis with generalized estimating equations (GEE) give strong support for the assumption, for example, that physical activity during adolescence and young adulthood is an important determinant of maximal aerobic power at the age of 27, and that this relationship is not merely a result of self-selection [9–11]. Tracking analyses show that physical activity [12] and dietary intake [13] have low stability and certainly lower than biologic factors such as overweight and serum cholesterol.

Motivation of the Participants: Adherence and Drop-Out

In order to motivate the participants to adhere to the longitudinal study, special measures were taken during the different age periods. During the adolescent period the physical measurements (anthropometry, physical fitness), completing questionnaires and interviews took place during regular school hours in classrooms and gymnasium, and in the purpose-built mobile research unit parked in front of the school buildings. The main reason for dropout was leaving school (because of the parents moving house and/or selection of the pupil by the school authorities). The dropout percentage of 24% was therefore foreseen.

After 1985, the participants had left school and were spread out over the country. They were therefore asked to continue their participation by visiting the laboratories in Amsterdam for one whole day. The dropout percentages were 14% in 1985, 9% in 1991, and 11% in 1993. Selective dropout was investigated by testing differences in the relevant characteristics between those who continued to participate and those who dropped out of the study.

From the start, the participants were continuously informed by booklets reporting the general results of the AGAHLS and their personal records. Moreover, comparisons were made of their own personal results with the mean values of the entire longitudinal group and, if possible, with the age- and sex-specific norms of the entire Dutch population.

PhD Theses Produced

Since the 1993 measurements, three PhD theses have been published, making use of the longitudinal database of the AGAHLS and demonstrating the importance of such a longitudinal study for health-related research. Dr. Jos W.R. Twisk studied the tracking of blood cholesterol over a 15-year period and its relationship with other risk factors for coronary heart disease, and developed a new methodological approach [14]. Tracking analysis shows the stability of a certain risk factor over time and/or the predictability of future values by early measurements. A new method was applied to calculate tracking coefficients, based on a statistical model in which the initial value of the variable of interest is related to the entire longitudinal development of the same variable. The standard regression coefficient related to the initial value can be interpreted as a tracking coefficient [15]. The parameters of the model are estimated with GEE, a method which is suitable for the longitudinal analysis of both continuous and dichotomous outcome variables. Comparison of the GEE-tracking coefficients with more traditional methods revealed that the latter mainly underestimates the real tracking phenomenon. In addition to tracking analyses, further analyses were performed to determine the factors influencing the tracking of cholesterol and HDL [16], and the longitudinal relationship between life-style and biological risk indicators for CVD [17–19], between personality characteristics and risk indicators for CVD [20] and between life-style and lung function parameters was studied [21].

Dr. Desiree C. Welten studied the calcium intake in relation to bone status during youth [22]. Her thesis focused on the problems encountered in measuring dietary calcium intake longitudinally by means of the cross-check dietary history method. Furthermore, she analyzed the relationship between calcium intake and (peak) bone mass, measured with Dual Energy X-ray Absorptiometry (DEXA) in the lumbar spine. Three research questions were formulated: (a) Is there a relationship between calcium intake during youth and the development of peak bone mineral density when the influence of physical activity and body weight was accounted for [23]? (b) How well does the calcium and dairy intake track from adolescence into adulthood? (c) Is a newly developed dairy questionnaire a valid method to recall the calcium intake of 8 and 16 years previously in 29-year-old males and females [24, 25]? The main conclusion was that no significant effects of the calcium intake were found. However, a meta-analysis seems to provide overall evidence that 1% bone mass loss per year can be prevented in premenopausal females by a calcium supplementation of 1,000 mg/day [26]. The calcium and dairy intake track only modestly, and these intakes during adolescence seem to be relatively poor predictors for adult values. In young adults, the retrospectively reported calcium intake seems to be a relatively poor estimation of the actual calcium intake of 8–16 years ago.

Dr. Frank J. van Lenthe described the development of a central pattern of body fat from adolescence into adulthood [27]. On the basis of the literature it was speculated that not only total body fatness (as measured with the sum of 4 skinfolds), but also its distribution over the body (as measured by trunk-extremity skinfold ratios) is related to risk factors for cardiovascular diseases [28]. Between the mean ages of 13 and 29 years, the trunk-extremity skinfold ratios remain relatively constant in females, but a marked increase is found in males. The magnitude of the longitudinal tracking coefficient of 0.55 suggests that the roots of a central pattern of body fat in adulthood are already present in the teens [29]. The influence of the timing of biological maturation on the development of a central pattern of body fat showed that only girls with a relatively early menarche have significantly higher trunk-extremity skinfold ratios between 13 and 27

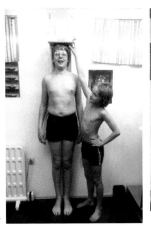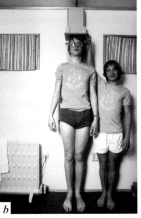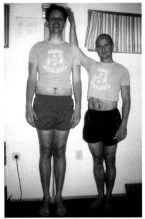

a   *b*   *c*

Fig. 4. Growth and development of two subjects from pictures made at ages 13(a), 17(b) and 32(c).

years of age, than relatively late menarcheal girls [30]. Behavioral variables (such as activity, nutrient intake, smoking and alcohol consumption) did not affect the development of a central pattern of body fat in this age-period [31]. However, type A behavior, after adjustment for total body fatness, was significantly negatively correlated at the age of 27 (in both sexes) and the personality traits 'dominance' and 'rigidity' were significantly negatively correlated between 13 and 21 years of age (only in males) with trunk-extremity skinfold ratios [32].

Van Mechelen et al. [33] reported a significant longitudinal relationship between resting heart rate, on the one hand, and CVD risk indicators (blood pressure and maximal oxygen uptake) on the other hand. These relationships did not change substantially when corrected for smoking and physical activity.

Third Period (1995–1999): The Amsterdam Growth and Health Longitudinal Study: A Model for Health Promotion?

In 1996 and 1997, follow-up measurements were completed in approximately 450 participants at the mean age of 32 (fig. 4). Not only the participants in the longitudinal group were included, but for the second time also the participants in the control group, who were measured once during their teenage period.

There were two reasons for including the control group: the first reason was to increase the number of participants in this cohort study in order to compensate for the inevitable drop-out that occurred in the previous 20–25 years, and to retain a minimal number of participants for statistical analyses of the longitudinal data. The second, more important reason, was to answer the following research question: Do repeated measurements and knowledge of the results between the ages of 12 and 34 years in the longitudinal sample, compared to the control sample with only two repeated measurements (one during adolescence and one at the age of 32), exert beneficial effects on the development of the health status? The results can be subdivided into three categories:

(1) The effects on nine biological risk factors for chronic diseases were limited: in men a borderline significant difference was found in the 20-year change for the body fat distribution (ratio of subscapular and triceps skinfold, S/T ratio), favoring the longitudinal group [34]. A significantly healthier effect was seen in systolic blood pressure in the control group. In women only the change in S/T ratio was better in the intervention group.

(2) The effect on dietary intake was also relatively small: out of the 14 nutrients the longitudinal group showed a significantly larger decrease in the mono- and disaccharides only, as compared to the control group [35].

(3) Contrary to the hypothesis that repeated medical check-ups combined with health information should increase the level of daily physical activity, both males and females in the control group showed a significantly smaller decrease in physical activity compared to the longitudinal group [36].

Last Period (2000–2004)

In 2000, a ninth repeated measurement took place, in which a non-invasive measurement was also included to estimate pre-clinical atherosclerosis of blood vessels in collaboration with Prof. C.D.A. Stehouwer (Department of Internal Medicine of the VU University Medical Center), measurement of heel bone by ultrasound (Dr. P.T.A.M. Lips), and retrospective measurement of birth-weight in collaboration with Prof. H.A. Delemarre-van de Waal. Collaboration has also been established with the Erasmus University Medical Center in Rotterdam (Department of Internal Medicine). Genetic markers of obesity (Prof. S.W.J. Lamberts) and osteoporosis (Prof. H.A.P. Pols) will be measured in the DNA of venous blood that has been collected from the participants in the past.

Five other research questions to be addressed in this period are:

- What is the importance of life-style factors (physical activity, dietary intake, alcohol consumption and smoking) for the development of biological CVD risk indicators over a period of 23 years in males and females between the ages of 12 and 36?
- What is the relative importance of relevant life-styles during adolescence and (young) adulthood for the bone mineral density of males and females in their thirties?
- What is the influence of biological risk indicators for CVD (lipoproteins, blood pressure, body fat, aerobic fitness), life-style risk indicators for CVD (nutrient intake, physical activity, alcohol consumption and smoking) and their interaction on early preclinical atherosclerosis?

- Is there a relationship between birth weight and the development of biological and life-style risk factors (between 12 and 36 years of age) and indicators of osteoporosis and atherosclerosis at the age of 36?
- What is the relationship between coffee consumption and subjectively experienced health, and what is the role of claimed sensitivity in this relationship?

In 2002, Dr. Lando L.J. Koppes finished his PhD thesis on alcohol consumption [37]. He showed the development of alcohol consumption from adolescence into adulthood: in women of all age groups, wine is the most popular alcoholic beverage, while men prefer beer. The mean amount of alcohol consumed peaks at age 21 in men (13.5 units per drinker per week) and in women at age 36 (9.1 units per drinker per week) [38].

The relationships of alcohol consumption with serum cholesterol [39] revealed that 32-year-old participants who consumed more than 10 alcoholic drinks per week have more favorable HDL-cholesterol levels compared with non-drinkers. From the relationship between alcohol consumption and personality characteristics [40] it was concluded that alcohol consumption was significantly associated with lower personality scores with regard to social inadequacy, rigidity and self-sufficiency. The validity of measurement of alcohol by a quantity-frequency questionnaire (QFQ) and/or a cross-check dietary history interview (DHI), revealed that (1) overall greater alcohol consumption was reported using DHI, and (2) the precision and validity of the QFQ appeared to be low [41].

In the year 2002, two supplements were published with data from the AGAHLS. First, the *International Journal of Sports Medicine* published a supplement entitled 'The relationship between physical activity and physical fitness in youth and cardiovascular health later in life, what longitudinal studies can tell' [42, 43]. Included are research papers from several longitudinal studies with three papers from the AGAHLS [44–46]. Second, a supplement was published in the journal *Bone*, entitled 'Mechanical loading of bone, bridging the gap between animal and human studies' [46, 47]. Included is an AGAHLS-paper about the relationship between physical activity and bone mass [49].

In 2003, Dr. Claire M. Bernaards published her thesis about smoking behavior. She found that the prevalence of smoking over the 20-year period increased gradually in both sexes, and that biological maturation, whether measured as skeletal age, or as years from peak height velocity, or as years from menarche (in women) is not a better predictor of smoking during adolescence than calendar age [50]. The relative validity of instruments to measure life-time smoking behavior was estimated by comparing retrospectively with prospective calculated pack-years over a period of 23 years (between 13 and 36 years

public health problem is impending. This problem requires effective public policy responses [14]. Given the high prevalence of overweight in many countries, and the environmental (nongenetic) nature of the problem, there is considerable potential for risk reduction. Although long-term changes of life-style behaviors like dietary intake and physical activity are hard to achieve in children and adults, the result of improved lifestyle behaviors will be the prevention and retardation of severely negative effects on the health and wellbeing of individuals and societies.

In order to be able to cope with the pediatric problem to prevent adult disease, it is important to get a better picture of the early risk factors and preventive factors for later disability and disease, and to understand the pathways through which these factors result in the health effects at adult age. This knowledge could result in improved identification of persons who are at high risk for later disease, and it could target interventions and be of help in monitoring the effects of interventions. Importantly, it could even explain why certain interventions are effective and others are not.

Prospective Observational Research

Most of the information needed for adequate prevention cannot be gathered using experimental study designs because of ethical restrictions, and neither with retrospective research because of the high risk of recall bias. Luckily, there is increasing awareness of the necessity of prospective observational research. In 1995 an update was given on an inventory of ongoing European longitudinal studies in the behavioral and medical sciences [15]. From the large of number studies (215) that minimally had three time points of measurements of at least 30 subjects over a minimum of 3 years of follow-up one may presume that many studies worldwide must have gathered information on the early predictors of adult health. However, the list of such studies becomes relatively small when only a few inclusion criteria are sharpened (table 1).

Table 1 gives an overview of prospective observational longitudinal studies in general populations. The overview is restricted to those studies with at least 8 years of follow-up in 100 subjects, covering measurements of lifestyles *and* biological risk-factors for chronic diseases assessed from adolescence into young adulthood (i.e. covering at least the age range from 17 to 21 years). Only studies that published about the relationships between lifestyle and biological risk factors are included. The studies were found through a search in the above-mentioned inventory of European longitudinal studies, and through a MEDLINE search performed on 27 February 2003 on the Title/Abstract words '(child* OR adolescen*) AND ((adult AND age) OR adulthood) AND

Table 1. Overview of longitudinal studies on lifestyle and health from adolescence into adulthood

Name of the study	Country	Measurements period	n	Participants age range	gender	n at start–end	a	b	c	d	e	f	g	h	i	j	Key publications
Amsterdam Growth and Health Longitudinal Study	The Netherlands	1977–2000	9	13–36	M & F	600–375	X	X	X	X	X	X	X	X	X	X	[16–17]
Cardiovascular Risk in Young Finns Study	Finland	1980–1992	5	3/18–15/30	M & F	3,596–2,370	X	X	X	X	X		X	X	X	X	[19–21]
Children in the Community Study	USA	1983–1991	3	14–22	M & F	776–644			X	X	X				X	X	[22, 23]
Danish Youth and Sports Study	Denmark	1983–1991	2	17–25	M & F	305–203	X		X	X	X	X	X	X			[24, 25]
Dunedin Multidisciplinary Health and Development Study	New Zealand	1975–1998	10	3–26	M & F	1,037–930	X	X	X	X	X	X	X		X	X	[26, 27]
Leuven Longitudinal Study on Lifestyle, Fitness and Health	Belgium	1969–1996	9	13–40	M	588–166	X	X	X	X	X	X	X	X	X	X	[28, 29]
Muscatine Study	USA	1971–1999	8	8–42	M & F	14,066–725	X		X	X	X	X	X		X	X	[30–32]
Northern Finland 1966 Birth Cohort	Finland	1980–1997	2	14–31	M & F	11,399–8,767	X	X	X	X	X	X			X	X	[33, 34]
Northern Ireland Young Hearts Project	Northern Ireland	1989–1999	3	12–22	M & F	1,015–508	X	X	X	X	X	X	X	X	X	X	[35, 36]
Québec Family Study	Canada	1980–1992	2	13–25	M & F	790–151	X		X	X	X		X		X		[37–39]
'Swedish Activity and Fitness Study'	Sweden	1974–1992	2	16–34	M & F	425–278	X		X	X	X	X	X		X	X	[40, 41]

a = Physical activity; b = dietary intake; c = alcohol consumption; d = tobacco smoking; e = anthropometry; f = indicators of physical fitness; g = cardio-vascular disease risk-factors (blood pressure, and/or cholesterol); h = indicators of bone health; i = other indicators of health status; j = psychological/sociolog-ical characteristics.

(lifestyle OR alcohol OR tobacco OR smoking OR (physical AND activity) OR diet) AND (longitudinal OR follow OR cohort)', followed by reference checking of potentially relevant articles, and a search for other publications from authors who wrote about a potentially relevant cohort.

Description of the Included Studies

Eleven studies that met our inclusion criteria were identified. Table 1 indicates for each study, the name, country, period and number of measurements, the age range, gender and number of participants, the measured variables, and key publications. The common feature of these studies is that they prospectively investigated the relationships between lifestyle behaviors and health characteristics over the important life transition from adolescence into adulthood. Inevitably, these studies differ with respect to volume, quality, scope, accomplishments, and promise. In addition to the summary in table 1, these studies will now be discussed in alphabetic order.

The Amsterdam Growth and Health Longitudinal Study (AGAHLS), started as a 4-year mixed longitudinal study focussing at the growth, physical activity and fitness of teenagers [16]. None of the first and second year pupils from the two participating secondary schools refused to attend a first measurement at adolescence. About 35% dropped out over the following 23 years. The participants from one school were asked to attend all nine measurements while those from the other school attended a maximum of one measurement at adolescence plus the two last measurements at the ages of 32 and 36 years [see chapter by Kemper et al., pp 167–182]. The measured variables *a* through *g* and *j* in table 1 have been assessed at each measurement, and in addition to the listed variables, birth weight and arterial wall properties are important other measured variables in the AGAHLS.

The Cardiovascular Risk in Young Finns Study is a collaborative effort of all university departments of pediatrics and several other institutions in Finland to study the risk factors of coronary heart disease (CHD) and their determinants in children and adolescents. Boys and girls in the wide age range from 3–18 years were included in the first measurement in 1980. The attrition rate was about 34% over the 12 years of follow-up. In addition to articles on the development with age and the inter-relations of the assessed CHD risk factors, main articles are published on socioeconomic status, and clustering and tracking of CHD risk factors.

The focus of the Children in the Community Study was on the prevalence and risk factors for psychiatric symptoms in late childhood and adolescence. The randomly sampled participants were sons and daughters of women who had been interviewed 11 years before the start of this study. Given the focus on psychiatric disorders, and demographic and other psychosocial variables, it is not surprising that physical activity, diet, and several aspects of health that are assessed in the other summarized studies were not assessed here.

The Danish Youth and Sports Study is a relatively small school-based study. Only two-thirds of the initial population of 305 adolescent boys and girls attended the second measurement 8 years later. Published articles mainly focus at physical activity, fitness, and other CHD risk factors.

The Dunedin Multidisciplinary Health and Development Study consists of an unselected sample of boys and girls born between April 1972 and March 1973 in one hospital in New Zealand. The large number of publications on the birth cohort involve studies on birth weight, psychosocial aspects, problem behavior, dental health and diverse other aspects of health.

The Leuven Longitudinal Study on Lifestyle, Fitness and Health is the only included study that did not involve assessments in females. The 588 boys who were followed longitudinally were selected on pragmatic grounds from an original cross-sectional sample in 1969 of 4,278 boys. Like the AGAHLS, it is a school-based study involving children from entire classes which was initially designed to provide information of the natural growth, physical activity and fitness of teenagers. Other variables like bone mineral density, stress and coping have been added at adult age.

The Muscatine Study is a population-based investigation of cardiovascular disease risk factors. It was originally designed as a cross-sectional school-based study. The initial follow-up measurements were performed only in the boys and girls who at that time were still at those schools. This resulted in the large attrition of participants. Although smoking and alcohol consumption have been assessed, practically all publications on lifestyle involve physical activity. Some other variables used in the Muscatine Study are fasting insulin and glucose, left-ventricular mass, carotid intima-media thickness and coronary artery calcium.

Investigations in the Northern Finland 1966 Birth Cohort started with lifestyle, biological and sociological measurements of the mothers of the cohort members in the 6th month of their pregnancy. The information obtained here was linked with perinatal and later outcomes obtained from measurements by the study group at ages of 14 and 31 years, and obtained from national registers. A large diversity of variables, like social economic status, oral health habits, hormones, criminal behavior, mental disorders, and neurological handicaps have formed the basis of publications. No data are available on adolescent dietary intakes, whereas the number of publications on adolescent physical activity, tobacco and alcohol use is small.

In order to search for causes of the high death rates from CHD in Northern Ireland, the Young Hearts Project was initiated. The original survey was completed in boys and girls from 16 randomly sampled representative schools of secondary education. About 50% of the original cohort participated in the last measurement so far at the age of 22 years. Not surprisingly, most publications on the Project are about the socioeconomic, lifestyle and biological risk factors for CHD (including birth weight), whereas a few publications on adult age bone mineral status are available.

The Québec Family Study is designed to investigate genetic and environmental influences on several biochemical, physical and physiological characteristics. Together with their parents, the participants were recruited using the local media. The participants were 8–18 years of age at the time of the first measurement. Only a few of the many publications on the Québec Family Study involved the longitudinal data from adolescence into adulthood.

The participants in the 'Swedish Activity and Fitness Study' were randomly selected pupils of randomly selected schools that were geographically and rural/urban representative, and of both practical and theoretical programs. Most publications on this study are about physical activity and/or fitness while one publication is about neck, shoulder and low back symptoms.

Conclusions

Given the increase in the number of elderly people in Western countries and the increases in certain risk factor levels for later chronic diseases, a public health problem with important economic repercussions is foreseen. Increased attention to the need for primary prevention and early detection of people at risk for chronic diseases is needed together with evidence-based preventive actions. Because lifestyle is expected to be one of the most important predictive factors for the occurrence of disease later in life, finding ways to improve it is one of our major present challenges. Hopefully, the studies outlined in this chapter, together with other studies will develop the knowledge that will result in a change in the minds of policy makers and the public from a relatively passive state of short-term thinking to a more proactive state to prevent (costs of) disease.

References

1   Van Oers JAM: Gezondheid op Koers? Volksgezondheid Toekomst Verkenning. Houten, Bohn Stafleu Van Loghum, 2002.
2   Stampfer MJ, Hu FB, Manson JE, Rimm EB, Willett WC: Primary prevention of coronary heart disease in women through diet and lifestyle. N Engl J Med 2000;343:16–22.
3   Daviglus ML, Liu K, Greenland P, Dyer AR, Garside DB, Manheim L, Lowe LP, Rodin M, Lubitz J, Stamler J: Benefit of a favorable cardiovascular risk-factor profile in middle age with respect to Medicare costs. N Engl J Med 1998;339:1122–1129.

4   Curhan GC, Willett WC, Rimm EB, Spiegelman D, Ascherio AL, Stampfer MJ: Birth weight and adult hypertension, diabetes mellitus, and obesity in US men. Circulation 1996;94:3246–3250.

5   Curhan GC, Chertow GM, Willett WC, Spiegelman D, Colditz GA, Manson JE, Speizer FE, Stampfer MJ: Birth weight and adult hypertension and obesity in women. Circulation 1996;94:1310–1315.

6   Barker DJ, Godfrey KM, Fall C, Osmond C, Winter PD, Shaheen SO: Relation of birth weight and childhood respiratory infection to adult lung function and death from chronic obstructive airways disease. BMJ 1991;303:671–675.

7   Yarbrough DE, Barrett-Connor E, Morton DJ: Birth weight as a predictor of adult bone mass in postmenopausal women. Osteoporos Int 2000;11:626–630.

8   Must A, Jacques PF, Dallal GE, Bajema CJ, Dietz WH: Long-term morbidity and mortality of overweight adolescents: A follow-up. N Engl J Med 1992;327:1350–1355.

9   Srinivasan SR, Myers L, Berenson GS: Predictability of childhood adiposity and insulin for developing insulin. Diabetes 2002;51:204–209.

10   Gunnell DJ, Frankel SJ, Nanchahal K, Peters TJ, Davey Smith G: Childhood obesity and adult cardiovascular mortality: A 57-year follow-up study based on the Boyd Orr cohort. Am J Clin Nutr 1998;67:1111–1118.

11   Bentley JR, Ferrini RL, Hill LL: American College of Preventive Medicine public policy statement: Folic acid fortification of grain products in the US to prevent neural tube defects. Am J Prev Med 1999;16:264–267.

12   Troiano RP, Flegal KM, Kuczmarski RJ, Campbell SM, Johnson CL: Overweight prevalence and trends for children and adolescents. The National Health and Nutrition Examination Surveys, 1963 to 1991. Arch Pediatr Adolesc Med 1995;149:1085–1091.

13   de Onis M, Blossner M: Prevalence and trends of overweight among preschool children in developing countries. Am J Clin Nutr 2000;72:1032–1039.

14   Dietz WH, Bland MG, Gortmaker SL, Molloy M, Schmid TL: Policy tools for the childhood obesity epidemic. J Law Med Ethics 2002;30:83–87.

15   Zentralstelle für Psychologische Information und Dokumentation der Universität Trier. Inventory of European longitudinal studies in the behavioral and medical sciences – Update 1990–1994. Trier, ZPID, University of Trier, 1995.

16   Kemper HCG: Growth, Health and Fitness of Teenagers: Longitudinal Research in International Perspective. Basel, Karger, 1985.

17   Kemper HCG: The Amsterdam Growth Study: A Longitudinal Analysis of Health, Fitness and Lifestyle. Champaign, Human Kinetics, 1995.

18   Akerblom HK, Viikari J, Kouvalainen K: Cardiovascular risk factors in Finnish children and adolescents. Acta Paediatr Scand Suppl 1985;318:5–212.

19   Akerblom HK, Viikari J, Raitakari OT, Uhari M: Cardiovascular Risk in Young Finns Study: General outline and recent developments. Ann Med 1999;31(suppl 1):45–54.

20   Raitakari OT, Porkka KV, Taimela S, Telama R, Rasanen L, Viikari JS: Effects of persistent physical activity and inactivity on coronary risk factors in children and young adults. The Cardiovascular Risk in Young Finns Study. Am J Epidemiol 1994;140:195–205.

21   Valimaki MJ, Karkkainen M, Lamberg-Allardt C, Laitinen K, Alhava E, Heikkinen J, Impivaara O, Makela P, Palmgren J, Seppanen R, et al: Exercise, smoking, and calcium intake during adolescence and early adulthood as determinants of peak bone mass. Cardiovascular Risk in Young Finns Study Group. BMJ 1994;309:230–235.

22   Cohen P, Cohen J: In Mahwah NJ (ed): Life Values and Adolescent Mental Health. New York, Lawrence Erlbaum, 1996.

23   Cohen P, Cohen J, Kasen S, Velez CN, Hartmark C, Johnson J, Rojas M, Brook J, Streuning EL: An epidemiological study of disorders in late childhood and adolescence. I. Age- and gender-specific prevalence. J Child Psychol Psychiatry 1993;34:851–867.

24   Andersen LB, Henckel P, Saltin B: Maximal oxygen uptake in Danish adolescents 16–19 years of age. Eur J Appl Physiol Occup Physiol 1987;56:74–82.

25   Andersen LB, Haraldsdottir J: Tracking of cardiovascular disease risk factors including maximal oxygen uptake and physical activity from late teenage to adulthood: An 8-year follow-up study. J Intern Med 1993;234:309–315.

26 Silva PA: The Dunedin Multidisciplinary Health and Development Study: A 15 year longitudinal study. Paediatr Perinat Epidemiol 1990;4:76–107.
27 Silva PA, Stanton WR: From child to adult: The Dunedin Multidisciplinary Health and Development Study. Auckland, New Zealand. London, Oxford University Press, 1996.
28 Beunen GP, Malina RM, Van't Hof MA, Simons J, Ostyn M, Renson R, Van Gerven D: Adolescent Growth and Motor Performance: A Longitudinal Study of Belgian Boys. Champaign, Human Kinetics, 1988.
29 Lefevre J, Philippaerts R, Delvaux K, Thomis M, Claessens AL, Lysens R, Renson R, Vanden Eynde B, Vanreusel B, Beunen G: Relation between cardiovascular risk factors at adult age, and physical activity during youth and adulthood: The Leuven Longitudinal Study on Lifestyle, Fitness and Health. Int J Sports Med 2002;23(suppl 1):S32–S38.
30 Lauer RM, Connor WE, Leaverton PE, Reiter MA, Clarke WR: Coronary heart disease risk factors in school children: The Muscatine study. J Pediatr 1975;86:697–706.
31 Lauer RM, Lee J, Clarke WR: Factors affecting the relationship between childhood and adult cholesterol levels: The Muscatine Study. Pediatrics 1988;82:309–318.
32 Clarke WR, Woolson RF, Lauer RM: Changes in ponderosity and blood pressure in childhood: the Muscatine Study. Am J Epidemiol 1986;124:195–206.
33 Rantakallio P: The longitudinal study of the northern Finland birth cohort of 1966. Paediatr Perinat Epidemiol 1988;2:59–88.
34 Tammelin T, Nayha S, Hills AP, Jarvelin MR: Adolescent participation in sports and adult physical activity. Am J Prev Med 2003;24:22–28.
35 Gallagher AM, Savage JM, Murray LJ, Davey Smith G, Young IS, Robson PJ, Neville CE, Cran G, Strain JJ, Boreham CA: A longitudinal study through adolescence to adulthood: the Young Hearts Project, Northern Ireland. Publ Hlth 2002;116:332–340.
36 Boreham C, Savage JM, Primrose D, Cran G, Strain J: Coronary risk factors in schoolchildren. Arch Dis Child 1993;68:182–186.
37 Bouchard C: Genetic epidemiology, association, and sib-pair linkage: Results from the Québec Family Study; in Bray GA, Ryan DH (eds): Molecular and Genetic Aspects of Obesity. Baton Rouge, Louisiana State University Press, 1996, pp 470–481.
38 Campbell PT, Katzmarzyk PT, Malina RM, Rao DC, Perusse L, Bouchard C: Prediction of physical activity and physical work capacity (PWC150) in young adulthood from childhood and adolescence with consideration of parental measures. Am J Hum Biol 2001;13:190–196.
39 Katzmarzyk PT, Perusse L, Malina RM, Bergeron J, Bouchard C: Stability of indicators of the metabolic syndrome from childhood and adolescence to young adulthood: The Québec Family Study. J Clin Epidemiol 2001;54:190–195.
40 Barnekow-Bergkvist M, Hedberg G, Janlert U, Jansson E: Adolescent determinants of cardiovascular risk factors in adult men and women. Scand J Publ Hlth 2001;29:208–217.
41 Barnekow-Bergkvist M, Hedberg G, Janlert U, Jansson E: Prediction of physical fitness and physical activity level in adulthood by physical performance and physical activity in adolescence: An 18-year follow-up study. Scand J Med Sci Sports 1998;8:299–308.

Prof. Dr. Han C.G. Kemper
AGAHLS Research Group, Institute for Research in Extramural Medicine
VU University Medical Center
Van der Boechorststraat 7, NL–1081 BT Amsterdam (The Netherlands)
Tel. +31 20 4448407, Fax +31 20 4446775, E-Mail hcg.kemper.emgo@med.vu.nl

Kemper HCG (ed): Amsterdam Growth and Health Longitudinal Study.
Med Sport Sci. Basel, Karger, 2004, vol 47, pp 30–43

....
Longitudinal Data Analysis

Jos W.R. Twisk, Han C.G. Kemper

Institute for Research in Extramural Medicine (EMGO Institute),
VU University Medical Center (VUmc), Amsterdam, The Netherlands

Abstract

In this chapter, besides MANOVA for repeated measurements, two sophisticated methods to analyze longitudinal data are explained: generalized estimating equations (GEE) and
random coefficient analysis. All methods are illustrated with data from the Amsterdam
Growth and Health Longitudinal Study. Three variables (serum cholesterol, body fatness and
gender) measured nine times over a period of 23 years are used in the example in which five
research questions are answered: (1) What is the longitudinal development over time for
serum cholesterol? (2) Is there a difference in development of serum cholesterol between
males and females? (3) What is the stability of serum cholesterol? (4) What is the longitudinal relationship between serum cholesterol and body fatness? (5) Is the longitudinal relationship between serum cholesterol and body fatness different over time? GEE and random
coefficient analysis are suitable to answer all the above questions and are much more flexible
than MANOVA for repeated measurements.

Introduction

In the last 10 years, there has been a growing interest in longitudinal studies and in the statistical analysis of longitudinal data. Longitudinal studies are
defined as studies in which the outcome variable is repeatedly measured, i.e. the
outcome variable is measured in the same individual on several occasions. In
longitudinal studies the observations of one individual are not independent of
each other, they concern the same person. Therefore, statistical methods, which
assume independent observations, such as linear regression analysis and logistic
regression analysis, cannot directly be used in longitudinal studies. For data
analyses in longitudinal studies special statistical methods are developed, which
take into account that the repeated observations of each individual, are correlated [1–3]. The most traditional methods for analyzing longitudinal data are the

paired t test and (M)ANOVA for repeated measurements. With these methods, it is possible to investigate changes in a continuous outcome variable over time and to compare the development of a continuous outcome variable over time between different groups [4, 5]. In longitudinal research, however, there are many other questions to be answered (e.g. what is the relationship between the development of a continuous outcome variable and the development of (several) other variables?) and sometimes the longitudinal development of dichotomous or categorical outcome variables are of interest. In such (more complicated) situations, the paired t test or (M)ANOVA for repeated measurements can not be used. There are, however, other (more sophisticated) methods available that are suitable to answer these questions. In epidemiological studies, there are two such sophisticated methods frequently used, i.e. generalized estimating equations (GEE) [6, 7] and random coefficient analysis [8, 9]. Both methods are suitable for the analysis of the longitudinal relationship between a continuous outcome variable and several time-dependent and time-independent covariates. Furthermore, these methods are suitable for the longitudinal analysis of a dichotomous (or categorical) outcome variable in relation to the development of other variables [9–11]. Besides this, the sophisticated methods can also be used to analyze the stability (or tracking) of different variables over time [12]. The purpose of this chapter is to describe the different statistical methods available to analyze longitudinal data, and to illustrate these methods with an example based on data from the Amsterdam Growth and Health Longitudinal Study.

Materials and Methods

Dataset
The different statistical methods will be illustrated with a dataset with (only) three variables measured 9 times over a period of 25 years, i.e. serum cholesterol, body fatness (estimated by the sum of the thickness of four skinfolds, i.e. biceps, triceps, subscapular, and suprailiac, and which was expressed in cm), and gender. Table 1 shows descriptive information of the variables used in this example.

The research questions to be answered in this example are rather simple: (1) What is the longitudinal development over time for serum cholesterol? (2) Is there a difference in development in serum cholesterol over time between males and females? (3) What is the longitudinal relationship between serum cholesterol and body fatness? (4) Is the longitudinal relationship between serum cholesterol and body fatness influenced by gender? (5) Is the longitudinal relationship between serum cholesterol and body fatness different over time? (6) What is the stability or tracking for serum cholesterol over time?

To illustrate the differences between longitudinal analysis with continuous and dichotomous outcome variables, serum cholesterol was either expressed in mmol/l or was dichotomized in such a way that at each measurement the subjects with serum cholesterol values ≥ 5.2 mmol/l were classified in the 'risk' group. With the dichotomous outcome variable only research questions 3, 4, 5 and 6 will be answered.

Table 1. Descriptive information of the variables used in the example

Measurement	Age	Males/females	Serum cholesterol		Body fatness[1]
			continuous mmol/l	<5.2/≥5.2 %	
1	13	315/340	4.48 (0.74)	85/15	3.32 (1.41)
2	14	232/287	4.43 (0.69)	87/13	3.56 (1.54)
3	15	219/272	4.30 (0.73)	87/13	3.79 (1.71)
4	16	222/280	4.27 (0.75)	88/12	3.93 (1.74)
5	21	93/107	4.68 (0.79)	75/25	4.57 (1.93)
6	27	84/98	5.12 (0.93)	55/45	4.15 (1.59)
7	29	78/88	4.95 (0.85)	66/34	4.63 (1.92)
8	32	206/232	4.91 (0.86)	64/36	4.73 (1.92)
9	36	178/200	5.00 (0.92)	62/38	5.15 (1.80)

[1]Body fatness was operationalized by the sum of the thickness of four skinfolds (in 10 mm).

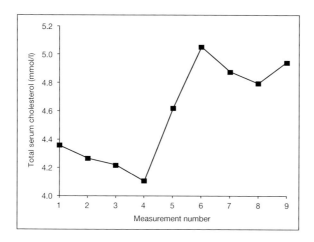

Fig. 1. Longitudinal development over time for serum cholesterol.

(1) What is the Longitudinal Development Over Time for Serum Cholesterol?
When there are only two measurements over time, the longitudinal development over time for a particular continuous outcome variable can be analyzed with the paired t test. When there are more than two measurements, (M)ANOVA for repeated measurements can be used. Figure 1 shows the development over time for serum cholesterol. With (M)ANOVA for repeated measurements, it was tested whether or not the change over time is statistically significant. The corresponding p value was <0.001.

Besides the fact that there is a significant change over time for serum cholesterol, figure 1 shows that the development over time is not really a linear one. With (M)ANOVA

Table 2. F ratios and p values of the (M)ANOVA for repeated measurements in order to answer the question what kind of development there is over time for serum cholesterol

Linear	Quadratic	Cubic
$F = 184.807$ ($p < 0.01$)	$F = 1.427$ ($p = 0.24$)	$F = 91.001$ ($p < 0.01$)

for repeated measurements, it is possible to answer the question: What kind of development over time is there for serum cholesterol? Table 2 shows the results of the corresponding (M)ANOVA for repeated measurements.

From table 2, it can be seen that the development can be (significantly) described by a linear function over time, as well as with a cubic function over time. However, according to the magnitude of the F ratio, the linear function describes the development over time more appropriate.

(2) Is There a Difference in Development in Serum Cholesterol Over Time between Males and Females?

The same statistical method (i.e. (M)ANOVA for repeated measurements) can be used when the development over time in a continuous outcome variable is compared between different groups. When this dichotomous independent variable is added to the (M)ANOVA for repeated measurements, basically three 'effects' can be estimated: (1) an overall time effect, i.e. is there a change over time in serum cholesterol for the total population? (2) An overall group effect, i.e. is there on average a difference in serum cholesterol between males and females? (3) a group by time interaction effect, i.e. is the change over time in serum cholesterol different for males and females?

Figure 2 shows the difference in development over time for males and females and table 3 shows the results of the (M)ANOVA for repeated measurements.

From table 3, it can be seen that there is an 'overall' time effect. This is not surprising, because that was already seen in the earlier analysis without gender. Furthermore, there is no significant 'overall' gender effect, but on the other hand there is a significant gender*time interaction. This indicates that on average, there is no difference between males and females, but that the development over time is different for males and females.

There are a few problems with the use of (M)ANOVA for repeated measurements. First of all, only complete cases are analyzed. This means that in the present example only 123 subjects are analyzed and that the information on many more subjects is ignored. Secondly, only continuous outcome variables can be analyzed and thirdly the independent variables can be either dichotomous or categorical, but cannot be continuous. In other words, it is attractive to use other methods to analyze the longitudinal data, which do not have the problems stated for (M)ANOVA for repeated measurements.

(3) What Is the Longitudinal Relationship between Serum Cholesterol and Body Fatness?

To answer the question whether there is an association between serum cholesterol and body fatness, (M)ANOVA for repeated measurements can not be used. In this situation, special sophisticated methods must be used. Within epidemiology, two sophisticated methods are mostly used, i.e. generalized estimating equations (GEE analysis) [6, 7] and

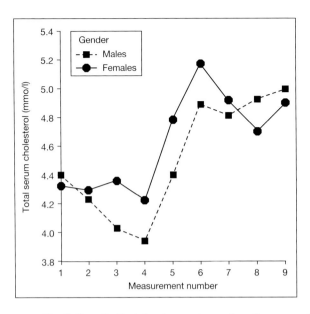

Fig. 2. Longitudinal development over time for serum cholesterol separate for males and females.

Table 3. F ratios and p values of the (M)ANOVA for repeated measurements in order to evaluate the development over time between males and females

'Overall' time effect	'Overall' gender effect	Gender*time interaction
F = 76.135; p < 0.001	F = 0.997; p = 0.32	F = 6.976; p < 0.001

random coefficient analysis, which is also known as multilevel analysis [8, 9]. Both methods are basically regression methods which takes into account the fact that the observations within one person are not independent. The difference between the methods is that they make this correction in a different way.

Within GEE, assuming (a priori) a certain 'working' correlation structure for the repeated measurements of the outcome variable [6, 7] does the correction for the dependency of observations. Depending on the software package used to estimate the regression coefficients, different correlation structures are available. They basically vary form an 'exchangeable' (or 'compound symmetry') correlation structure (i.e. the correlations between subsequent measurements are assumed to be the same, irrespective of the length of the interperiod) to an 'unstructured correlation structure'. In this structure no particular structure is assumed, which means that all possible correlations between repeated measurements has to be estimated.

The basic idea behind the use of random coefficient analysis in longitudinal studies is that the regression coefficients are allowed to differ between subjects. The simplest form of a random coefficient model in longitudinal studies is a model with just a random intercept, i.e. the baseline value is different for each subject (fig. 3a). It is also possible that the

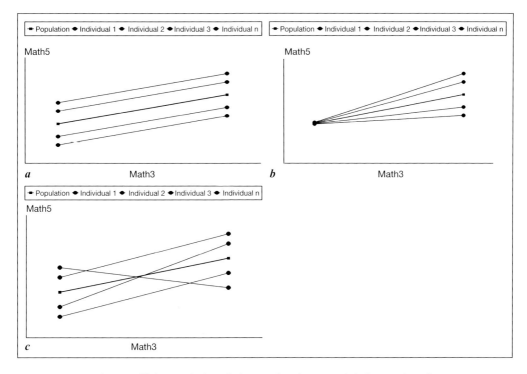

Fig. 3. Random coefficient analysis: *a* Only a random intercept. *b* Only a random slope with time. *c* Both a random intercept and a random slope with time.

intercept is not random, but that the regression coefficient with time is considered to be random (i.e. random slope). In other words, the development of a certain variable over time is allowed to vary among individuals (fig. 3b). The most interesting possibility is the combination of a random intercept and a random slope with time (fig. 3c). Of course it is also possible to consider the regression coefficients of the other predictor variables to be random. However, that situation will not be considered in this example.

Besides the fact that the development of different variables can be related to each other, the main advantages of using either GEE analysis or random coefficient analysis is that all longitudinal data are used in the analysis (irrespective of the number of repeated measurements). Furthermore, the time-period between subsequent measurement can be unequal and can be different for different individuals, and for both methods the outcome variable can be continuous as well as dichotomous.

Firstly, both methods are used to analyze the longitudinal relationship between serum cholesterol as a continuous outcome variable and body fatness, and, secondly, the same relationship was analyzed for serum cholesterol as a dichotomous outcome variable.

Continuous Outcome Variable

Table 4 shows the results of the GEE analysis and the random coefficient analysis to answer the question whether there is a longitudinal relationship between serum cholesterol and body fatness.

Table 4. Regression coefficients, standard errors and p values of the GEE analysis and the random coefficient analysis in order to analyze the longitudinal relationship between serum cholesterol (as a continuous outcome variable) and body fatness

	Regression coefficient	SE	p value
GEE			
Exchangeable correlation	0.106	0.009	<0.001
Unstructured correlation	0.090	0.010	<0.001
Random coefficient analysis			
Random intercept	0.107	0.009	<0.001
Random intercept and slope	0.097	0.010	<0.001

Firstly, all four analyses reveal a highly significant longitudinal relationship between serum cholesterol and body fatness. Furthermore, it can be seen that both the regression coefficients and the standard errors of the regression coefficients (which are used to calculate the confidence intervals around the regression coefficient) are more or less the same for GEE and random coefficient analysis.

An important issue is the interpretation of the regression coefficient. What does it mean that the regression coefficient for body fatness is 0.106? Unfortunately, there is no straight-forward answer to that question. Basically, the regression coefficient estimated with a 'sophisticated' longitudinal data analysis (either GEE or random coefficient analysis) is a 'pooled' coefficient of a within-subject and a between-subject relationship. This has the following implication for the interpretation of the regression coefficients: suppose that for a particular subject the serum cholesterol concentration is relatively high at each of the repeated measurements and does not change much over time. Suppose further that for that particular subject body fatness is also relatively high at each of the repeated measurements. This indicates a longitudinal 'between-subjects' relationship between serum cholesterol and body fatness. Suppose that for another subject the serum cholesterol concentration increases rapidly along the longitudinal period, and suppose that for the same subject this pattern is also found for body fatness. This indicates a 'within-subject' relationship between serum cholesterol and body fatness. Both relationships are part of the overall longitudinal relationship, so both should be taken into account in the analysis of the longitudinal relationship. The regression coefficient estimated with either GEE analysis or random coefficient analysis 'combines' the two possible relationships into one regression coefficient. In other words, a longitudinal regression coefficient of 0.106 can indicate that a difference of 1 unit in body fatness between two persons is associated with a difference of 0.106 units in serum cholesterol, but can also indicate that in increase of one unit in body fatness within one person is associated with an increase of 0.106 units in serum cholesterol. The 'truth' will lie somewhere in between.

For GEE analysis we have analyzed the longitudinal data assuming two different correlation structures, i.e. an exchangeable correlation structure and an unstructured correlation structure. In the literature it is assumed that GEE analysis is robust against a wrong choice for a correlation structure, i.e. it does not matter which correlation structure is chosen, the results of the longitudinal analysis will not be very different [13, 14]. In this example, this is

Table 5. Interperiod correlation coefficients for serum cholesterol

	2	3	4	5	6	7	8	9
1	0.78	0.71	0.66	0.63	0.55	0.56	0.52	0.58
2		0.78	0.74	0.65	0.58	0.58	0.54	0.59
3			0.81	0.69	0.61	0.55	0.53	0.57
4				0.72	0.64	0.59	0.51	0.50
5					0.67	0.66	0.57	0.59
6						0.66	0.64	0.58
7							0.71	0.72
8								0.73

more or less true. There is not much difference between the results of an analysis with an exchangeable correlation structure and the results of an analysis with an unstructured correlation structure. This is, however, not always the case [14, 15]. In many situations, it is important to realize which correlation structure should be chosen for the analysis. One of the possibilities is to investigate the within-person correlation structure of the actual data and see which possible structure is the best approximation of the 'real' correlation structure. Furthermore, the simplicity of the correlation structure has to be taken into account. The number of parameters (in this case correlation coefficients) that needs to be estimated differs for the various working correlation structures. In the example dataset with nine repeated measurements, for instance, for an exchangeable correlation structure only one correlation coefficient has to be estimated, while for the unstructured correlation structure, 36 correlation coefficients must be estimated. As a result, the power of the statistical analysis is influenced by the choice for a certain structure. The best option is therefore is to choose the simplest structure that fits the data well. So, the first step in choosing a certain correlation structure can be to investigate the within-person correlation coefficients for the outcome variable (table 5). Based on these coefficients, an exchangeable correlation structure seems to be the simplest most appropriate choice in this particular situation.

For random coefficient analysis, one has to choose which coefficients have to be assumed random. This choice is easier than the choice for a working correlation structure in GEE analysis. This is due to the fact that most standard software, which can be used for random coefficient analysis, provides -2 log likelihood values of each model, which can be used to evaluate different models. In the present example, a model with both a random intercept and a random slope with time was found to be the most appropriate, although the magnitude of the regression coefficient and the standard error were not much influenced by this choice. However, comparable to what has been said for GEE analysis, also for random coefficient analysis, the choice for allowing different regression coefficients to be random can have an impact on the magnitude of the regression coefficient and/or the standard error of the regression coefficient.

Dichotomous Outcome Variable
As been mentioned before, both GEE analysis and random coefficient analysis are suitable for the analysis of both continuous and dichotomous outcome variables. Table 6 shows

Table 6. Regression coefficients, standard errors and p values of the GEE analysis and the random coefficient analysis in order to analyze the longitudinal relationship between serum cholesterol (as a dichotomous outcome variable) and body fatness

	Regression coefficient	SE	p value
GEE			
Exchangeable correlation	0.243	0.029	<0.001
Unstructured correlation	0.204	0.029	<0.001
Random coefficient analysis			
Random intercept	0.363	0.049	<0.001
Random intercept and slope	0.357	0.051	<0.001

the results of both methods in answering the question whether there is a longitudinal relationship between serum cholesterol (dichotomized with a cut-off value of 5.2 mmol/l) and body fatness.

As for the analysis with a continuous outcome variable, body fatness was highly related to serum cholesterol. Also comparable to the analysis with a continuous outcome variable, there was not much difference between the GEE analysis with an exchangeable correlation structure and GEE analysis with an unstructured correlation structure and there was not much difference between the two random coefficient analyses. The most interesting finding is the difference between GEE analysis and random coefficient analysis. Both the regression coefficients and the standard errors were remarkably higher when estimated with random coefficient analysis compared to GEE analysis. Although this looks strange, it not really is. It is important to realize that the regression coefficient calculated with GEE analysis is the average value of the individual regression lines. Therefore, the regression coefficients estimated with GEE analysis are called 'population averaged' [3, 6]. The regression coefficients calculated with random coefficient analysis can be seen as the 'average individual' or 'subject specific'. Figure 4 illustrates this difference for an analysis with a continuous outcome variable (i.e. linear longitudinal regression analysis) and for the analysis with a dichotomous outcome variable (i.e. logistic longitudinal regression analysis) with only a random intercept. For the linear longitudinal regression analysis, both the GEE and the random coefficient approach leads to the same results, i.e. the 'population average' coefficient is equal to the 'subject specific' coefficient. For the logistic longitudinal regression analysis, both approaches lead to different results. This has to do with the fact that in logistic regression analysis the intercept has a different interpretation than in linear regression analysis. From figure 4, it can be seen that the regression coefficients calculated with a logistic GEE analysis will always be lower than the coefficients calculated with a comparable random coefficient analysis [16–18]. This was also seen in the results reported in table 6.

The interpretation of the regression coefficients is exactly the same as has been mentioned for continuous outcome variables; i.e. the regression coefficient reflects both the 'between-subjects' relationship and the 'within-subject' relationship. In the analysis with dichotomous outcome variables, however, the regression coefficients are mostly transformed to odds ratios (EXP[regression coefficient]).

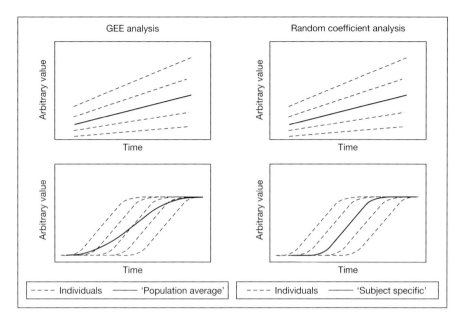

Fig. 4. Differences between GEE analysis and random coefficient analysis for a continuous and dichotomous outcome variable.

GEE Analysis or Random Coefficient Analysis?

Both GEE- and random coefficient analyses are highly suitable to analyze longitudinal data, because in both methods a correction is made for the dependency of the observations within one individual. The question than arises: Which of the two methods is better? Unfortunately, no clear answer can be given. For continuous outcome variables, GEE analysis with an exchangeable correlation structure is the same as a random coefficient analysis with only a random intercept. The correction for the dependency of observations with an exchangeable 'working correlation' structure is the same as allowing individuals to have random intercepts. When the dependency of observations is slightly more complicated, GEE analysis with a different correlation structure can be used or random coefficient analysis with additional random regression coefficients for other variables (e.g. time). Although random coefficient analysis is slightly more flexible, it should be realized that 'regular' random coefficient analysis is limited by the fact that the random regression coefficients are assumed to be normally distributed with mean zero.

When a dichotomous outcome variable is analyzed in a longitudinal study, should GEE analysis or random coefficient analysis be used? If one is performing a population study such as the AGAHLS, and one is interested in the relationship between a dichotomous outcome variable and several predictor variables, GEE analysis will probably provide the most 'valid' answer. However, if one is interested in the individual development over time of a dichotomous outcome variable, random coefficient analysis will probably provide the most 'valid' results. It should, however, also be noted that random coefficient analyses with a dichotomous outcome variable are not fully developed yet. Different software packages give different

Table 7. Regression coefficients, standard errors and p values of the GEE analysis (with an exchangeable correlation structure) in order to analyze the longitudinal relationship between serum cholesterol (as a continuous outcome variable) and body fatness separately for males and females

	Regression coefficient	SE	p value
Males	0.190	0.014	<0.001
Females	0.062	0.011	<0.001

results and within one software package there is (mostly) more than one possibility to estimate the coefficients and, unfortunately, the different estimation procedures often led to totally different results [15]. In other words, although in theory random coefficient analysis can be suitable in some situations, in practice one should be very careful in using this method in the longitudinal analysis of a dichotomous outcome variable.

(4) Is the Longitudinal Relationship between Serum Cholesterol and Body Fatness Influenced by Gender?

Another advantage of using either GEE analysis or random coefficient analysis in the analysis of longitudinal data is that both methods are regression methods. This implies that all possibilities available in 'normal' linear or logistic regression analysis are also available for the longitudinal regression methods. For example, it can be investigated whether the observed relationship between serum cholesterol and body fatness is influenced by gender, or in other words, is gender an effect modified or a confounder. As in 'normal' regression analysis, effect modification is easily investigated by adding an interaction term between gender and body fatness to the model. In all analysis, the interaction was highly significant with a negative sign, indicating that the relationship between serum cholesterol and body fatness was stronger for males (coded as 1) than for females (coded as 2). Because there is a significant interaction with gender, separate results should be reported for males and females. Table 7 shows the results of a GEE analysis with a continuous outcome variable and an exchangeable correlation coefficient performed for males and females separately.

Because of the separate regression coefficients for males and females, the question whether or not gender is a confounder in the longitudinal relationship between serum cholesterol and body fatness is no longer an issue. However, suppose that the interaction was not significant, then the next step is to investigate whether or not gender is a confounder in the relationship between serum cholesterol and body fatness. This can be investigated by reanalyzing the data with gender added to the model. The magnitude of the change in regression coefficient for body fatness between the model with gender and the model without gender will give an indication of the 'confounding effect' by gender.

(5) Is the Longitudinal Relationship between Serum Cholesterol and Body Fatness Different Over Time?

Another question, which can be of importance, is whether or not the longitudinal relationship between serum cholesterol and body fatness is different over time. Because this basically means that one is interested in the interaction between time and body fatness, the question can be easily answered by adding the interaction between time and body fatness to the longitudinal regression models. When this is done in the present example a significant interaction with a positive sign was found. This means that the positive relationship between serum cholesterol and body fatness is stronger when time increases, i.e. it means that the relationship between serum cholesterol and body fatness is stronger at the end of the longitudinal period.

(6) What is the Stability or Tracking of Serum Cholesterol Over Time?
In the epidemiological literature, tracking is used to describe the relative stability of the longitudinal development of a certain variable. There is no single widely accepted definition of tracking, but the following concepts are involved: (1) the relationship (correlation) between early measurements and measurements later in life, or the maintenance of a relative position within a distribution of values in the observed population over time, and (2) the predictability of future values by early measurements [19, 20]. The most traditional way of analyzing tracking of a continuous outcome variable is estimating the correlation coefficient between a baseline measurement and a follow-up measurement. This is especially suitable in a longitudinal study with two measurements, but the more repeated measurements available, the more complicated it will be to use the correlation coefficient to evaluate tracking over time. An alternative way is to use one of the sophisticated methods to analyze the relationship between the initial value of the variable of interest and the total development of that variable over time. The standardized regression coefficient of the initial value can then be interpreted as a 'longitudinal' correlation coefficient.

The traditional way of analyzing tracking of a dichotomous outcome variable is to calculate the proportion of subjects who are in a 'high' risk group at baseline and who maintain their position in the 'high' risk group at the follow-up measurement. Like for the continuous outcome variables, this approach is suitable for longitudinal studies with only two measurements. When there are more than two measurements, longitudinal logistic regression analysis can be used to estimate the relationship between 'risk' group status at baseline and the development of that status during follow-up. As a result of this longitudinal logistic regression analysis an odds ratio can be calculated, which expresses the magnitude of tracking for 'high' risk subjects, i.e. what is the odds for subjects who are in the 'high' risk group at baseline to maintain 'at risk' over time, compared to the odds to be 'at risk' over time for the subjects who were not 'at risk' at baseline.

Table 8 shows both tracking coefficients for serum cholesterol. For the example, in both situations separate tracking coefficients were calculated for males and females.

Although it is difficult to interpret the magnitude of the tracking coefficients [20], it seems that both coefficients reveal moderate-to-high tracking for serum cholesterol over the total longitudinal follow-up period of 25 years.

Conclusion

Several methods are available to analyze longitudinal data. The most simple methods (i.e. (M)ANOVA for repeated measurement) can only be used to answer rather 'simple' research questions and has some major disadvantages. Sophisticated statistical methods (i.e. GEE analysis and random coefficient

Table 8. Tracking coefficients and 95% confidence intervals (estimated with GEE analysis with an exchangeable correlation structure) for serum cholesterol (both as a continuous and dichotomous outcome variable) separately for males and females

	Tracking coefficient[1]	95% CI
Continuous outcome variable		
Males	0.57	0.46–0.68
Females	0.56	0.49–0.63
Dichotomous outcome variable		
Males	6.60	3.36–12.94
Females	11.91	6.50–21.80

[1] For continuous outcome variables, standardized regression coefficients were estimated and for dichotomous outcome variables odds ratios.

analysis) are suitable to answer almost all questions regarding longitudinal data, including the ones answered by (M)ANOVA for repeated measurements, and questions regarding stability or tracking. Furthermore, the sophisticated techniques are much more flexible. For continuous outcome variables, GEE analysis and random coefficient analysis are equally suitable, while for dichotomous outcome variables, GEE analysis seems to be the most appropriate sophisticated method.

References

1   Zeger SL, Liang K-Y: An overview of methods for the analysis of longitudinal data. Stat Med 1992;11:1825–1839.
2   Hand DJ, Crowder MJ: Practical Longitudinal Data Analysis. London, Chapman & Hall, 1996.
3   Diggle PJ, Liang K-Y, Zeger SL: Analysis of Longitudinal Data. New York, Oxford University Press, 1994.
4   Morrisson DF: Multivariate Statistical Methods. New York, McGraw-Hill, 1976.
5   Crowder MJ, Hand DJ: Analysis of Repeated Measures. London, Chapman & Hall, 1990.
6   Zeger SL, Liang K-Y: Longitudinal data analysis for discrete and continuous outcomes. Biometrics 1986;42:121–130.
7   Liang K, Zeger SL: Longitudinal data analysis using generalized linear models. Biometrica 1986; 73:45–51.
8   Laird NM, Ware JH: Random effects models for longitudinal data. Biometrics 1982;38:963–974.
9   Goldstein H: Multilevel Statistical Models, ed 2. London, Edward Arnold, 1995.
10 Vonesh EF, Carter RL: Mixed effect nonlinear regression for unbalanced repeated measures. Biometrics 1992;48:1–17.
11 Lipsitz SR, Laird NM, Harrington DP: Generalized estimating equations for correlated binary data: Using the odds ratio as a measure of association. Biometrika 1991;78:153–160.
12 Twisk JWR, Kemper HCG, van Mechelen W, Post GB: Tracking of risk factors for coronary heart disease over a 14 year period: A comparison between lifestyle and biological risk factors with data from the Amsterdam Growth and Health Study. Am J Epidemiol 1997;145:888–898.

13   Liang K-Y, Zeger SL: Regression analysis for correlated data. Annu Rev Publ Hlth 1993;14:43–68.
14   Twisk JWR: Different statistical models to analyze epidemiological observational longitudinal data: An example from the Amsterdam Growth and Health Study. Int J Sports Med 1997;18(suppl 3): S216–S224.
15   Twisk JWR: Applied Longitudinal Data Analysis for Epidemiology: A Practical Guide. Cambridge, Cambridge University Press, 2003.
16   Neuhaus JM, Kalbfleisch JD, Hauck WW: A comparison of cluster-specific and population-averaged approaches for analyzing correlated binary data. Int Stat Rev 1991;59:25–36.
17   Hu FB, Goldberg J, Hedeker D, Flay BR, Pentz MA: Comparison of population-averaged and subject specific approaches for analyzing repeated measures binary outcomes. Am J Epidemiol 1998;147:694–670.
18   Crouchley R, Davies RB. A comparison of GEE and random coefficient models for distinguishing heterogeneity, nonstationarity and state dependence in a collection of short binary event series. Stat Modeling 2001;1:271–285.
19   Ware JH, Wu MC: Tracking: Prediction of future values from serial measurements. Biometrics 1981;37:427–437.
20   Twisk JWR, Kemper HCG, Mellenbergh GJ: Mathematical and analytical aspects of tracking. Epidemiol Rev 1994;16:165–183.

Prof. Dr. Han C.G. Kemper
AGAHLS Research Group, EMGO Institute
VU University Medical Center
Van der Boechorststraat 7, NL–1081 BT Amsterdam (The Netherlands)
Tel. +31 20 4448407, Fax +31 20 4446775, E-Mail hcg.kemper.emgo@med.vu.nl

Kemper HCG (ed): Amsterdam Growth and Health Longitudinal Study.
Med Sport Sci. Basel, Karger, 2004, vol 47, pp 44–63

....

Longitudinal Trends, Stability and Error of Biological and Lifestyle Characteristics

Lando L.J. Koppes, Jos W.R. Twisk, Han C.G. Kemper

Institute for Research in Extramural Medicine (EMGO Institute),
VU University Medical Center (VUmc), Amsterdam, The Netherlands

Abstract

Background/Aims: Describing individual trends in time, and estimating stability, tracking and error are advantages of longitudinal research. The AGAHLS has extensive data to exploit these advantages. *Methods:* Graphs of the lifestyle behaviors physical activity, energy intake, alcohol and tobacco use, and the biological characteristics Body Mass Index (BMI), sum of four skinfolds (S4S), systolic and diastolic blood pressure (SBP and DBP), total cholesterol (TC), high-density lipoprotein cholesterol (HDL-C), and aerobic fitness (VO_2max) are given for the men and women followed from age 13 to 36 years. The stability and error of these variables are assessed. *Results:* The mean value of most biological characteristics worsened with the rising age of the population. Stability of most variables increased with age, and was higher for the biological than the lifestyle characteristics. Error was higher in the lifestyle behaviors. *Conclusion:* The large diversity in the development, stability and error of characteristics has implications for research and (lifestyle) interventions.

Despite numerous advantages, longitudinal research has its shortcomings. The internal validity of longitudinal research is threatened by learning and testing effects, while its external validity is threatened by cohort and period effects [1]. Within the AGAHLS the magnitude of these types of bias over the first 4 years of the study was investigated through the use of a mixed longitudinal design [2], and over the first 19 years through the re-inclusion of the participants from the Purmerend school [see chapter by Kemper et al., pp 5–7]. Fortunately, the amount of bias, overall, was not as large as expected. Other shortcomings or difficulties of longitudinal research are its limitation in disentangling the effects of age and period, (selective) attrition of participants, the necessary retention of long-term faculty and staff, and the relatively high costs involved.

Despite its shortcomings, longitudinal research has much to offer. First, it is less susceptible to cohort effects than cross-sectional research, so that longitudinal studies are preferable when the main goal is to understand changes on an individual level [2]. Second, longitudinal studies are superior in revealing the longitudinal relationships between the development of one factor with the development of another factor, for example, revealing how the development of lifestyle factors such as physical activity, dietary intake, alcohol consumption or tobacco smoking, coincides with the development of biological factors such as body composition, blood pressure, serum cholesterol or aerobic fitness [3]. Third, longitudinal studies are most suitable in uncovering the modification of these relationships with age. To give an example of age modification; in adolescence and young adulthood the relationship between the consumption of alcohol and all-cause mortality is linear, while in middle-aged and elderly people a U-shaped relationship exists [4, 5]. Fourth, longitudinal studies are needed to show the impact of changes in lifestyles, or psychological characteristics, on aspects of health [6]. Fifth, longitudinal research is able to depict the associations between data recorded at young ages and the occurrence of disease later in life [7]. Finally (although not being exhaustive on the merits of longitudinal research), longitudinal studies have the potential to explore the tracking and stability of a characteristic [8].

This last-mentioned opportunity with longitudinal research, quantification of the stability of a characteristic over time is important from a public health perspective because it is an important factor in the effectiveness of lifestyle interventions to improve health. If the stability of a characteristic is very high, the level of this characteristic is usually hard to change, and interventions that focus on this characteristic are predestined to be ineffective. On the other hand, interventions that focus on characteristics that do not track very well are more likely to be effective. However, this effect on an unstable characteristic will probably be short-lived. Knowledge of the level of tracking of a characteristic further helps to answer the question whether or not lifestyle interventions should be given to the whole population or to a sub-sample. If stability is high, the value of a characteristic is a good predictor for the value of this characteristic later in life. Therefore, in such a case it is prudent to focus interventions on those with unhealthy scores, because the risk that the others will attain unhealthy scores is low. On the other hand, if stability is extremely low, it will be better to focus on the whole group.

In this chapter, we describe the development of the most important lifestyle and biological factors that have been measured longitudinally in the

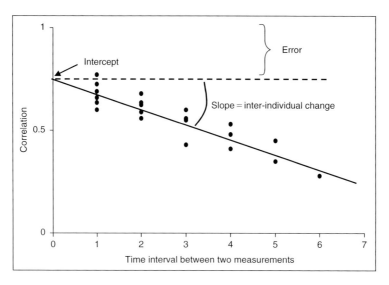

Fig. 1. Graphical description of inter-period correlation matrix (after Veling and Van 't Hof [9]).

AGAHLS over the whole 23-year follow-up period. Secondly, a description is given of the development of the concordance between two measurements of these factors that are several years apart. It will be shown that this concordance between two measurements is often different in adolescence than in adulthood. Third, a description is given of the stability and the test-retest irreproducibility (error) of these lifestyle and biological characteristics. Stability and error are estimated with techniques that are modifications of the method developed by Van 't Hof et al. (see ref. [9] for a description), which uses a matrix of inter-period correlation coefficients (IPCs, see fig. 1). It has been shown that the magnitude of the IPCs may be approximated by a linear function of the time interval between two measurements [10]. The intercept is the theoretical correlation coefficient between two measurements with an inter-period equal to zero years, and may be interpreted as the test-retest reproducibility. One minus the intercept is the test-retest irreproducibility (or error). The slope of the line, or the decay in correlation per year increase of the measurement interval, is interpreted as the interindividual change over time of the measured characteristic in question. Unfortunately, the magnitude of the slope is confounded by the amount of error because the slope depends on the height of the intercept. Variables with low test-retest reliability (small intercept) are less likely to have a steep slope. In this chapter a new technique is proposed to calculate a measure of stability that controls for the fact that variables with low test-retest reliability are less likely to have a steep slope. The resulting estimate is ideal to compare the stability of different variables.

Methods

Lifestyle Behaviors and Biological Characteristics
The lifestyle behaviors studied in this chapter are habitual physical activity (expressed in metabolic equivalents; METs), tobacco smoking (g/day), alcohol consumption (g/day), and dietary energy intake (kJ/kg bodyweight). Physical activity was assessed using a face-to-face interview, and was calculated as the intensity of performed activities times the duration of those activities. Activities of less than 4 METs were not taken into account. Tobacco smoking was assessed using a questionnaire, while alcohol consumption and dietary energy intake were assessed using a face-to-face interview. In the last measurement, in the year 2000, dietary energy intake and physical activity were measured with a computerized version of the face-to-face interviews [11].

The biological characteristics that have been measured longitudinally over the whole 23 years of AGAHLS follow-up are body mass index (BMI), sum of four skinfolds (S4S), systolic and diastolic blood pressure (SBP and DBP), serum total and high-density lipoprotein cholesterol (TC and HDL-C), and the maximal oxygen uptake per kg bodyweight (VO_2max).

Analyses
Gender-controlled inter-period partial correlation coefficients for all used variables were calculated. These coefficients give an indication of the combination of interindividual change over time and error. The coefficients are close to one if interindividual change and error are low. The coefficients are close to zero if interindividual change and error are high. The coefficients were calculated for the five age periods from 13 to 16 years, 16 to 21, 21 to 27, 27 to 32, and 32 to 36 years. These correlation coefficients, thus, indicate the relative concordance between two assessments that are, respectively, 3, 5, 6, 5, and 4 years apart. In addition, these correlation coefficients were calculated for the four longer measurement intervals between the assessments at the ages of 13 and 21 years, 16 and 27, 21 and 32, and 27 and 36 years. In all partial correlation coefficients, only the data from the 130 participants who attended all measurements were taken into account. This has the advantage that differences in the results between age periods are not caused by differences in subpopulations.

Stability estimates that are not confounded by the level of error were calculated by dividing the inter-period correlation coefficient of a long period (e.g. 13 to 21) by the average of the coefficients of the separate periods it contains (13 to 16 and 16 to 21). With this method, stability estimates were calculated for four periods of 8 to 11 years. The mean of these four estimates gives an indication of the average stability over the 23-year period. In addition, error estimates are calculated as follows:

$$\text{Error} = 1 - [\text{mean } r_{(1\text{period})} + (\text{mean } r_{(1\text{period})} - r_{(2\text{periods})})],$$

where r is the partial inter-period correlation coefficient. Analogous to the stability estimates, errors were estimated for four periods of 8 to 11 years. The mean of these four errors gives an indication of the average error in the measurement of a variable over the 23-year period.

Finally, a graphic representation of the decrease in predictability in time of the value of a characteristic from a previous measurement of that characteristic will be given for the

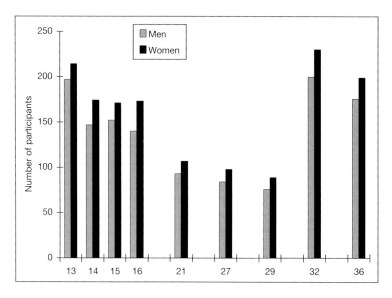

Fig. 2. Number of participants at different ages at measurement.

lifestyle behaviors and the biological characteristics. In these graphs, the error is represented by the intercept deviation from the value 1, and the slope relative to the height of the intercept represents the stability.

Results

The number of male and female participants at the different years of measurement is depicted in figure 2. Descriptive data of the lifestyle behaviors are shown in figures 3 through 8. The amount of physical activity decreased with age, especially during adolescence in boys. The increased physical activity levels at age 36 are caused by the change in assessment method from the face-to-face method to the computerized method [12]. In the computerized method more low-intensity activities have been recorded. Dietary energy intake per kg bodyweight decreased with age as well. With respect to alcohol consumption, a rise with age in the number of drinkers, and in the amount of consumption per drinker was seen. The percentage smokers and the amount of tobacco smoked increased until the age of 21 years, and have decreased since then.

Descriptive data of the biological characteristics are shown in figures 9 through 17. Over the 23 years of follow-up, BMI of the AGAHLS participants has shown a dramatic increase of about $7 \, kg/m^2$. In line with the BMI increase, the sum of four skinfolds increased with an average of 1.6 cm. The decrease

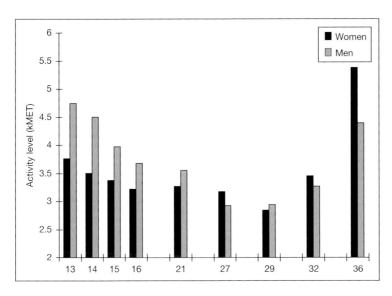

Fig. 3. Mean habitual physical activity level at the different ages at measurement.

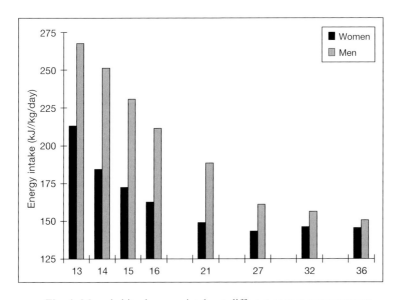

Fig. 4. Mean habitual energy intake at different ages at measurement.

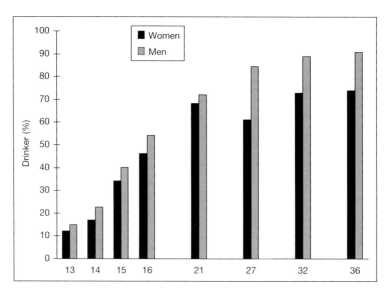

Fig. 5. Percentages of male and female participants who were at least occasional consumers of alcohol at different ages at measurement.

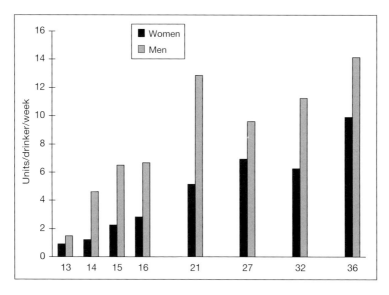

Fig. 6. Mean alcohol intake per drinker at different ages at measurement.

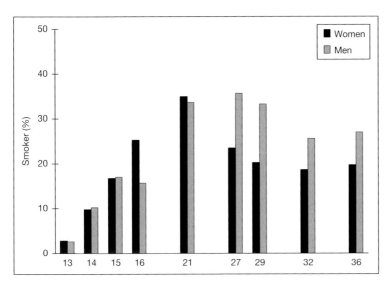

Fig. 7. Percentages of male and female participants who smoked tobacco at different ages at measurement.

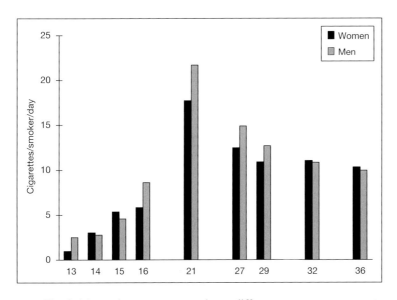

Fig. 8. Mean tobacco use per smoker at different ages at measurement.

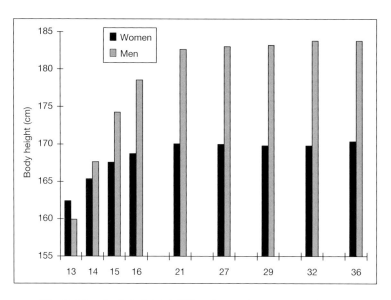

Fig. 9. Mean body height at different ages at measurement.

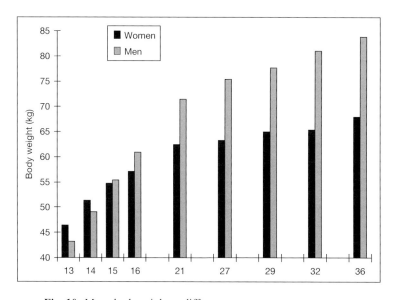

Fig. 10. Mean bodyweight at different ages at measurement.

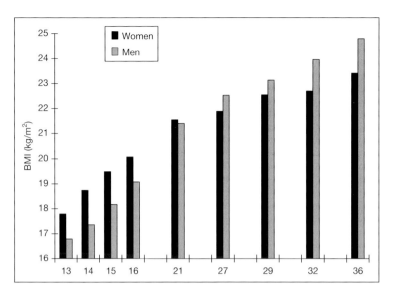

Fig. 11. Mean Body Mass Index (BMI) at different ages at measurement.

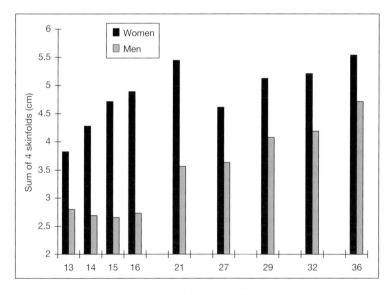

Fig. 12. Mean sum of four skinfolds at different ages at measurement.

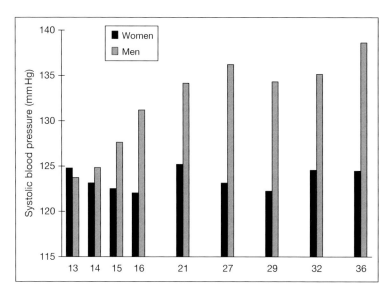

Fig. 13. Mean systolic blood pressure at different ages at measurement.

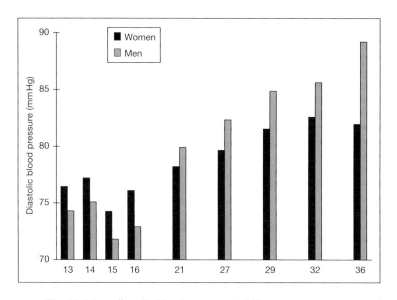

Fig. 14. Mean diastolic blood pressure at different ages at measurement.

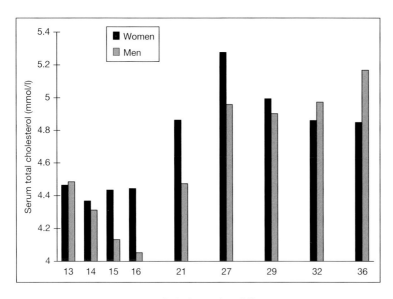

Fig. 15. Mean serum total cholesterol at different ages at measurement.

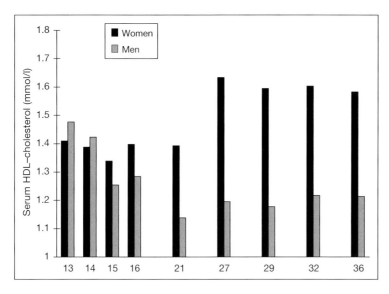

Fig. 16. Mean serum high-density lipoprotein cholesterol (HDL-C) at different ages at measurement.

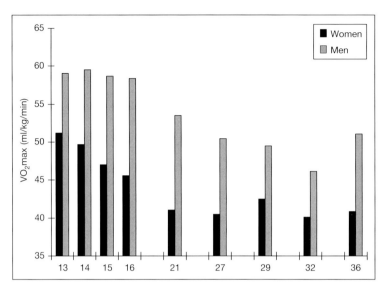

Fig. 17. Mean maximum oxygen uptake per kg bodyweight (VO$_2$max) at the different ages at measurement.

observed in women between the ages of 21 and 27 years is probably due to a change in observer. The observer measuring until the age of 21 years overestimated the thickness of the skinfolds relative to the observer measuring from the age of 27 years onwards. In men SBP increased over the 23 years of follow-up, while in women, it remained almost stable. In contrast, DBP increased in both men and women, although, more in men than women. TC increased in both men and women, while HDL-C decreased in men, but increased in women. VO$_2$max decreased an average of almost 10 ml/kg/min.

The results of the inter-period partial correlation analyses of the lifestyle behaviors are shown in table 1. For alcohol and tobacco consumption, strong increases in the magnitude of the correlation coefficients were found with age. To a smaller degree, and only from the 8- to 11-year intervals, this increase in the concordance between two measurements with rising age was found for physical activity and energy intake as well. Correlation coefficients of energy intake were higher than those of physical activity.

Table 2 shows the inter-period partial correlation coefficients for the biological characteristics. These correlation coefficients are higher than those found in table 1 for the lifestyle behaviors. This was especially true for BMI, S4S, and TC, where the 3- to 6-year period correlation coefficients were >0.7. Although less obvious than the coefficients for the lifestyle behaviors, increases

Table 1. Partial correlation coefficients of lifestyle behaviors measured 3–6 years apart (***A***), and 8 to 11 years apart (***B***) in 130 participants who all attended each of these 6 measurements

	Physical activity METs	Energy intake kJ/kg	Alcohol g/day	Tobacco g/day
A				
13→16	0.39	0.59	0.21	0.11
16→21	0.32	0.47	0.20	0.52
21→27	0.28	0.58	0.38	0.65
27→32	0.34	0.70	0.64	0.54
32→36	0.31	0.65	0.73	0.71
Mean	0.33	0.60	0.43	0.51
B				
13→21	0.12	0.28	0.08	0.19
16→27	0.15	0.39	0.21	0.52
21→32	0.21	0.59	0.50	0.31
27→36	0.26	0.56	0.58	0.58
Mean	0.19	0.46	0.34	0.40

Table 2. Partial correlation coefficients of biological characteristics measured 3 to 6 years apart (***A***), or 8 to 11 years apart (***B***) in 130 participants who all attended each of these 6 measurements

	BMI	S4S	SBP	DBP	TC	HDL-C	VO$_2$max
A							
13→16	0.82	0.79	0.48	0.40	0.74	0.60	0.51
16→21	0.73	0.66	0.52	0.54	0.74	0.59	0.67
21→27	0.74	0.67	0.72	0.66	0.68	0.67	0.49
27→32	0.83	0.77	0.49	0.52	0.68	0.68	0.55
32→36	0.88	0.80	0.58	0.55	0.74	0.81	0.63
Mean	0.80	0.74	0.56	0.53	0.72	0.67	0.57
B							
13→21	0.60	0.54	0.43	0.36	0.66	0.57	0.40
16→27	0.59	0.51	0.49	0.50	0.69	0.49	0.36
21→32	0.66	0.60	0.45	0.38	0.67	0.65	0.55
27→36	0.72	0.70	0.63	0.55	0.61	0.70	0.64
Mean	0.64	0.59	0.50	0.45	0.66	0.60	0.49

Table 3. Stability estimates of lifestyle behaviors and biological characteristics for four periods of follow-up measurements, and the average stability over the four periods

		13→21	16→27	21→32	27→36	Mean
Lifestyle	Physical activity	0.33	0.51	0.68	0.80	0.58
behaviors	Energy intake	0.53	0.75	0.91	0.82	0.75
	Alcohol	0.38	0.43	0.99	0.85	0.66
	Tobacco	0.61	0.88	0.52	0.92	0.73
Biological	BMI	0.77	0.80	0.85	0.84	0.82
characteristics	S4S	0.75	0.76	0.83	0.89	0.81
	SBP	0.86	0.79	0.75	1.16	0.89
	DBP	0.76	0.83	0.64	1.02	0.81
	TC	0.89	0.98	0.99	0.87	0.93
	HDL	0.96	0.78	0.97	0.94	0.91
	VO_2max	0.68	0.63	1.05	1.08	0.86

Stability estimate = Partial correlation coefficients of 2 periods/average of the partial correlation coefficients of the underlying 2 periods.

For example: Stability estimate$_{13→21}$ = $r_{13→21}/(0.5*(r_{13→16} + r_{16→21}))$, where the r's are the partial inter-period correlation coefficients of depicted in tables 1 and 2.

with age in the concordance between successive measurements were found for most biological characteristics.

Table 3 shows that the stability in time of the lifestyle behaviors is smaller than that of the biological characteristics. Highest stability was found for TC (0.93), and lowest for physical activity (0.58). As for the correlation coefficients of tables 2 and 3, most stability estimates increased with rising age. For SBP, DBP and VO_2max, stability estimates larger than one were found. Stability estimates larger than one are not plausible theoretically, however, because of measurement error they are possible. Stability estimates larger than one are more likely in variables with high stability and relatively large measurement error. These two conditions were true for the three variables involved, as their mean stability estimates were ≥ 0.81, and their mean measurement errors were ≥ 0.35 (table 4). Measurement error was smallest for BMI (0.07), and largest for physical activity (0.54).

Figures 18 and 19 depict the predictability of the value of a characteristic from a previous measurement for the lifestyle behaviors and biological characteristics, respectively. The lines combine the mean stability and error estimates of tables 3 and 4. The error is represented by the difference between the intercept and one, while the slope (relative to the height of the intercept) represents the stability. Figure 18 shows that the predictability of the lifestyle behaviors

Table 4. Estimates of error in the measurement of lifestyle behaviors and biological characteristics for four periods of follow-up measurements, and the average error over the four periods

		13→21	16→27	21→32	27→36	Mean
Lifestyle behaviors	Physical activity	0.41	0.55	0.59	0.61	0.54
	Energy intake	0.22	0.34	0.30	0.20	0.27
	Alcohol	0.67	0.55	0.48	0.21	0.48
	Tobacco	0.56	0.35	0.12	0.32	0.34
Biological characteristics	BMI	0.05	0.12	0.10	0.02	0.07
	S4S	0.09	0.17	0.16	0.13	0.14
	SBP	0.43	0.25	0.24	0.55	0.37
	DBP	0.42	0.30	0.20	0.48	0.35
	TC	0.18	0.28	0.31	0.20	0.24
	HDL	0.38	0.24	0.31	0.21	0.29
	VO$_2$max	0.22	0.20	0.50	0.46	0.35

Error $= 1 - [\text{mean } r_{(1period)} + (\text{mean } r_{(1period)} - r_{(2periods)})]$, where the r's are the partial inter-period correlation coefficients depicted in tables 1 and 2.

For example: $\text{Error}_{13\to21} = 1 - [0.5*(r_{13\to16} + r_{16\to21}) + (0.5*(r_{13\to16} + r_{16\to21}) - r_{13\to21})]$.

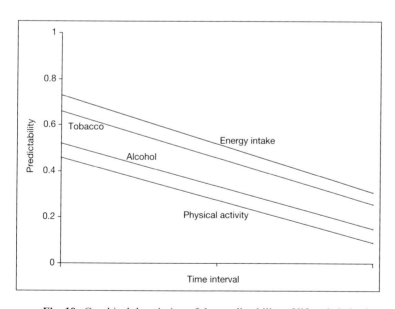

Fig. 18. Graphical description of the predictability of lifestyle behaviors.

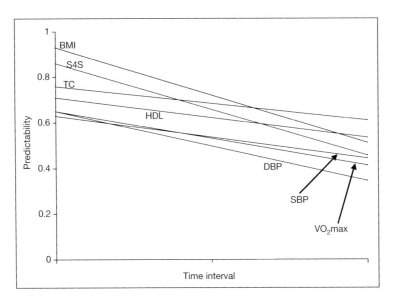

Fig. 19. Graphical description of the predictability of biological characteristics.

becomes very small with increasing time-interval. From figure 19, it can be concluded that the predictability of TC and HDL-C is better than that of BMI and S4S when the interval between measurements is large.

Discussion

Development

In this chapter, the development over 23 years of follow-up in the AGAHLS men and women of four lifestyle behaviors and seven biological characteristics is described. The percentage tobacco smokers was somewhat smaller, and that of alcohol drinkers (and >30 g/day drinkers) are somewhat higher than those in the general population [13–15]. Unfortunately, no other Dutch study used methods to assess habitual physical activity or dietary energy intake in a comparable way to the interviews that were used in the AGAHLS. The percentages of AGAHLS men and women at age 36 years with obesity (BMI >30) were 4 and 5% respectively, which is only 1–2% below the Dutch average. Percentages of AGAHLS men and women with TC levels above 6.5 mmol/l are, with 7 and 4%, slightly below average as well. The percentage of AGAHLS men with high blood pressure was equal to that of the general population, while that in AGAHLS women was somewhat smaller [13, 14].

Overall, it can be concluded, as far as comparisons are possible through the availability of equivalent data from other studies, that the AGAHLS population may be slightly healthier, but does not appear very different from the general Dutch population.

The mean values of most biological characteristics worsened with the rising age of the population. The two exceptions are SBP and HDL-C in women. Over the 23 years of follow-up hardly any change was seen for the mean SBP, and for HDL-C an improvement with age was seen. On the one hand, this is nothing new. These biological characteristics, which all are indicators of the risk of cardiovascular disease and mortality, simply worsen with aging. However, the magnitude of the deterioration is disturbing. For example, the percentage of the AGAHLS participants with overweight (BMI >25) has risen by 28% in only 15 years, from 6% at age 21 to 34% at the age of 36 years. Knowledge of the relationships between lifestyle behaviors and these biological risk-indicators for CVD is of major importance with regard to targeting health-improving lifestyle interventions. This kind of knowledge is being generated using AGAHLS data [see, for example, chapters by Snel et al., pp 123–131 and Kemper et al., pp 153–166].

Stability

In the introduction of this chapter we stated that certain stability estimates such as interperiod correlation coefficients are confounded by the amount of measurement error. We will now illustrate this statement with an example. The partial inter-period correlation coefficients of SBP we found were much smaller than those of BMI (means were 0.56, and 0.80, respectively). From this higher concordance between two BMI measurements one could conclude that the stability of BMI is higher than that of SBP. However, because of the larger error in the measurement of SBP, the opposite is true. The average stability of SBP was 0.89, while that of BMI was only 0.82.

The relatively simple stability estimate that is used here has a disadvantage as compared with the more intricate tracking estimates that are based on generalized estimating equations or on random coefficient analyses [see chapter by Twisk et al., pp 30–43]. This disadvantage is that not all available data are used, but only the data from those participants that attended all measurements. In contrast, the advantage of this is that the stability estimates of different variables or of different years of measurement are all based on the exact same participants. Thereby, differences in stability at different ages or between variables will not be confounded by differences in sub-samples of the population.

Highest stability was found for TC and HDL-C. This supposes a stronger inherited biological control over these parameters, than over the parameters for which lower stability coefficients were found (BMI, S4S, DBP, and VO_2max).

Changes in these latter parameters may therefore be more easily attained through changes in lifestyles. If the goal is to improve characteristics with high stability, like TC, HDL-C (and SBP), the interventions should be focused on those subjects with unhealthy values. This is because the subjects with unhealthy values will most likely hold these unhealthy values for a long period, while others are not very prone to worse values.

Dietary energy intake showed the highest stability of the four lifestyle behaviors, but still only 0.75. Physical activity was lowest, with 0.58. Values of these magnitudes presume that all four lifestyle behaviors are susceptible to interventions, but that the effects of interventions to improve the lifestyle behaviors are prone to be short-lived. Because of the lowest stability, this relatively poor durability of the intervention effects will be especially present for physical activity.

Error

Error was identified as one minus the estimated test-retest reliability (fig. 1). The amount of error was found high in the measurement of alcohol consumption, while it was even higher in the measurement of physical activity. Therefore, relationships with these variables are often doomed to remain not significant. True effects (or relationships) will have to be strong to be detected out of the large amount of noise. The biological characteristics overall showed less error than the lifestyle behaviors. Therefore, relationships with biological variables will more easily reach statistical significance. For the biological variables, the least measurement error was found for BMI and S4S, while the most error was found for SBP, DBP, and VO$_2$max. Analyses using these last three characteristics will therefore be less likely to result in significant findings compared with analyses using BMI or S4S. This difference is enlarged by the latter variables being less stable than the others, and therefore is more susceptible to change.

Conclusion

The rapid worsening in mean values of some biological characteristics with the rising age of the young and relatively healthy AGAHLS population raises concern for their health in the near future. The stability of many variables increases from adolescence into adulthood. Stability and error differ largely between the assessed variables. Stability was higher for the biological than the lifestyle characteristics (highest in TC and HDL-C, lowest in physical activity), while for error the opposite was true (lowest in BMI and S4S, and highest in physical activity). Especially in variables with high measurement error, tracking gives an underestimation of stability. The large diversity in the development, stability and error of lifestyle behaviors and biological characteristics has implications for the magnitude and statistical significance of inferential research findings, and the development and effectiveness of (lifestyle) interventions.

References

1   Van Mechelen W, Mellenbergh GJ: Problems and solutions in longitudinal research: From theory to practice. Int J Sports Med 1997;18:S238–S245.
2   Kemper HCG, Van 't Hof MA: Design of a multiple longitudinal study of growth and health in teenagers. Eur J Pediatr 1978;129:147–155.
3   Twisk JWR, Kemper HCG, Mellenbergh GJ, Van Mechelen W, Post GB: Relation between the longitudinal development of lipoprotein levels and lifestyle parameters during adolescence and young adulthood. Ann Epidemiol 1996;6:246–256.
4   White IR, Altmann DR, Nanchahal K. Alcohol consumption and mortality: Modeling risks for men and women at different ages. BMJ 2002;325:191.
5   Britton A, McPherson K: Mortality in England and Wales attributable to current alcohol consumption. J Epidemiol Community Health 2001;55:383–388.
6   Twisk JWR, Snel J, Kemper HCG, Van Mechelen W: Changes in daily hassles and life events and the relationship with coronary heart disease risk factors: A 2-year longitudinal study in 27–29-year-old males and females. J Psychosom Res 1999;46:229–240.
7   Twisk JWR, Van Mechelen W, Kemper HCG, Post GB: The relation between 'long-term exposure' to lifestyle during youth and young adulthood and risk factors for cardiovascular disease at adult age. J Adolesc Hlth 1997;20:309–319.
8   Twisk JWR, Kemper HCG, Mellenbergh GJ: Mathematical and analytical aspects of tracking. Epidemiol Rev 1994;16:165–183.
9   Veling SHJ, Van 't Hof MA: Data quality control methods in longitudinal studies; in Ostyn MG, Beunen G, Simons J (eds): Kinantropometry. Baltimore, University Park Press, 1980, pp 436–442.
10 Van 't Hof MA, Kowalski CJ: Analysis of mixed longitudinal data-sets; in Prahl-Andersen B, Kowalski CJ, Heyendael PHJM (eds): A Mixed Longitudinal Interdisciplinary Study of Growth and Development. New York, Academic Press, 1979, pp 161–172.
11 Kemper HCG, Koppes LL, De Vente W, Van Lenthe FJ, Van Mechelen W, Twisk JWR, Post GB: Effects of health information in youth and young adulthood on risk factors for chronic diseases-20-year study results from the Amsterdam growth and health longitudinal study. Prev Med 2002; 35:533–539.
12 Bakker I, Twisk JWR, Van Mechelen W, Mensink GB, Kemper HCG: Computerization of a dietary history interview in a running cohort: Evaluation within the Amsterdam Growth and Health Longitudinal Study. Eur J Clin Nutr 2003;57:394–404.
13 Van der Wilk EA: Introduction to the Compass. Volksgezondheid Toekomst Verkenning, Nationaal Kompas Volksgezondheid. Bilthoven, RIVM, 2003. http://www.nationaalkompas.nl
14 Blokstra A, Seidell JC, Smit AH, Bueno de Mesquita HB, Verschuren WMM: Morgen Project (in Dutch). Bilthoven, RIVM, 1997.
15 Swinkels H: Use of alcoholic beverages in the Netherlands: A comparison of some survey methods. Maandbericht Gezondheid (CBS) 1991;12:5–12.

Prof. Dr. Han C.G. Kemper
AGAHLS Research Group, Institute for Research in Extramural Medicine
VU University Medical Center
Van der Boechorststraat 7, NL–1081 BT Amsterdam (The Netherlands)
Tel. +31 20 4448407, Fax +31 20 4446775, E-Mail hcg.kemper.emgo@ med.vu.nl

Kemper HCG (ed): Amsterdam Growth and Health Longitudinal Study.
Med Sport Sci. Basel, Karger, 2004, vol 47, pp 64–77

....

Fetal Origins of Musculoskeletal and Cardiovascular Health at Adulthood

Saskia J. te Velde, Jos W.R. Twisk, Willem van Mechelen,
Han C.G. Kemper

Institute for Research in Extramural Medicine (EMGO Institute),
VU University Medical Center (VUmc), Amsterdam, The Netherlands

Abstract

Background: The fetal origins hypothesis proposes that impaired fetal growth is associated with risk factors for cardiovascular and musculoskeletal health. Fat-free mass (FFM) might be a link between these associations. We investigated whether birth weight was indeed associated with FFM and cardiovascular and musculoskeletal health, and subsequently whether FFM mediates these relationships. *Methods:* FFM, cardiovascular and musculoskeletal health were repeatedly measured in 335 subjects (27–36 years). Birth weight was obtained from a questionnaire. *Results:* Birth weight was positively associated with adult FFM and inversely with diastolic blood pressure (DBP) (in women), total cholesterol (TC) and the ratio between TC and serum HDL concentrations (TC:HDL). FFM as well as body weight, strengthen the associations. Furthermore, birth weight was associated with lumbar bone mineral content (BMC). *Conclusions:* In a young population, birth weight is indeed associated with FFM, and to DBP, TC, TC:HDL and BMC. These latter associations were mediated by FFM.

Background

The fetal origins hypothesis proposes that the intra-uterine period is critical for the development of several risk factors for chronic diseases, such as cardiovascular disease (CVD) and osteoporosis [1–4]. During the last decades, many papers have reported that lower birth weight is associated with raised blood pressure [5], and an increased risk for CVD later in life [4, 6–12]. Not much is known about the fetal origins of osteoporosis, however Gale et al. [13]

showed that birth weight was positively associated with bone area and bone mineral content (BMC) of the spine, femoral neck, and whole body.

More recently, Singhal et al. [14] suggested that the programming of lean body mass can be a link between birth weight, obesity and CVD. They observed a strong association between birth weight and fat free mass (FFM) in adolescents, but not between birth weight and fat mass (FM). The associations between birth weight and muscle mass later in life was also been reported by others [13, 15–17]. Unfortunately, they did not have data on risk factors for CVD, and were therefore not able to analyze whether FFM was really the link in the association between birth weight and risk factors for CVD. The association between birth weight and FFM might also be a link between birth weight and musculoskeletal health, since FFM is associated with bone density [18] and muscle strength [19].

In the Amsterdam Growth and Health Longitudinal Study (AGAHLS) data are available on body composition, cardiovascular health, and musculoskeletal health. Therefore, the aim of present study is to analyze whether or not in this population birth weight is related to body composition, cardiovascular and musculoskeletal health, and, subsequently, to study whether adult FFM is an mediator in the associations (if any) between birth weight and cardiovascular and musculoskeletal health.

Methods

Subjects and Design
Subjects were all participants of the AGAHLS which started in 1976 as an observational study. For the study presented here, the data from the last three repeated measurements, when the subjects had reached mean ages of 27, 33 and 36 years, were used. During all three measurements data were collected on body composition, cardiovascular and musculoskeletal health (fig. 1). At the mean age of 36 years, subjects filled in a questionnaire about their birth weight and gestational age.

Subjects were included in the analyses when they were born after 36 weeks, singleton and of Caucasian race. For the longitudinal analyses, 335 (198 women) had appropriate data on birth weight and at least one measurement of the outcome variable.

Birth Weight
Data on birth weight and gestation were obtained by a retrospective questionnaire. Most subjects retrieved information from a birth certificate, a birth announcement card or something similar (n = 237). Others used their parents as a source of information (n = 145), a method that has been proven to be valid [20–23]. Of the 382 subjects, 11 were twins, 27 were born before 37 weeks of gestation and another 9 subjects were non-Caucasian, and hence were excluded. Finally, the remaining 335 subjects all had at least one measurement on the outcome variables.

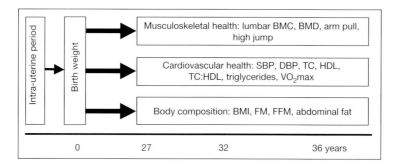

Fig. 1. Design of the study: the relationship between birth weight (as a measure of intra-uterine growth) and the different outcome measures: body composition, cardiovascular and musculoskeletal health.

Body Composition

As estimates for body composition were used, Body Mass Index (BMI), Fat mass (FM), abdominal fat (AF) and fat free mass (FFM).

BMI was calculated by dividing body weight (kg) by body height squared (m^2). Body weight (to the nearest 0.1 kg) and body height (to the nearest 0.001 m) were measured according to standard procedures [24], with subjects dressed only in underwear.

FM was calculated from the equations developed by Durnin and Womersley [25], which takes into account the thickness of the bicepital, tricepital, subscapular and suprailli-acal skinfolds. The thickness of these skinfolds were measured with a Harpenden skinfold calliper (Holtain, UK, van Rietschoten & Houwens, The Netherlands) according to standard procedures [24].

AF was estimated with the waist circumference [26] which was measured at umbilicus height with a flexible steel tape to the nearest 0.1 cm.

FFM was calculated by subtracting FM from the total body weight.

Cardiovascular Health

As estimates for cardiovascular health were used the systolic (SBP) and diastolic blood pressure (DBP), total serum cholesterol (TC) and HDL concentrations, the ratio between both (TC:HDL), triglyceride blood concentration, and cardiopulmonary fitness.

SBP and DBP were measured in sitting position with a sphygmomanometer (Speidl-Keller No. 2010; Franken & Itallie, The Netherlands) prior to a treadmill test. These pressures were measured twice and the lower values were recorded in mm Hg (with 5 mm Hg precision).

TC, HDL and TC:HDL were determined using venous blood with methods according to Huang et al. [27] and to Burnstein and Samaille [28]. The blood sampling and serum preparations were done between 08.30 and 12.30 h with subjects in a nonfasting state.

Cardiopulmonary fitness was operationalized as maximum oxygen uptake (VO$_2$max) relative to body weight and was expressed in $ml \cdot min^{-1} \cdot kg^{-2/3}$. VO$_2$max was measured by an open circuit method while running on a treadmill (Quinton, model 18–54, Lode BV, Groningen, the Netherlands) at 8 km/h and increasing slope, until exhaustion [29]. The Ergoanalyser (gasmeter, Mijnhardt BV, The Netherlands) continuously analyzed the collected expired air and printed the calculated VO_2 for each minute during the running test. The highest value was used as the maximum oxygen uptake (ml/min).

Musculoskeletal Health

Lumbar (L2–4) bone mineral content (BMC) and bone mineral density (BMD) were measured by dual X-ray absorptiometry (DEXA). The Norland XR 26 (Norland, Corp., Fort Atkinson, Wisc., USA) was used for the measurements at the mean ages of 27 and 32 years (first part of these measurements), and the Hologic QDR-2000 (S/N 2513; Hologic, Inc., Waltham, Mass., USA) at the mean ages of 32 years (second part of these measurements) and 36 years. In order to overcome differences in outcome caused by the changing of machines, standardized values (z-scores), separately for men and women and separately for year of measurement, were used.

Muscle strength was assessed by two physical fitness tests from the MOPER fitness test battery [30]: (1) Static arm pull: The subjects had two attempts to pull maximally with their best arm. Strength was measured (in kg) by a dynamometer (Bettendorff, Belgium), which was fixed to the wall in a way that the subject could pull horizontally. The best score was taken from the two obtained values. (2) Standing high jump: The subjects had to jump as high as possible twice (best score was used). They had to stand still on a plate, and were only allowed to bend their knees before jumping. The jumping height (in cm) was measured by a tape, which was fixed to a belt around their waist and the plate on the ground.

Statistical Analyses

Linear generalized estimating equations (GEE) analyses [31] were used to study the relationship between birth weight and the development of adult body composition (BMI, FM, AF and FFM), cardiovascular health indicators (SBP, DBP, TC, HDL, TC:HDL, tryglyceride blood concentration, VO_2max) and musculoskeletal health indicators (L-BMC, L-BMD, arm pull, high jump).

For the analyses two different models were used. A 'crude' model (model 1), which is only adjusted for sex and time of measurement. And a second model (model 2) was further adjusted for adult weight (as a time dependent co-variate).

In order to analyze the possible mediating effect of FFM, FFM was added in a statistical model which already included birth weight, time of measurement and sex. The change in the regression coefficient for birth weight between the two models was used as a measure of mediating effect.

Furthermore, it was investigated whether sex was an effect modifier in the all studied associations. If the interaction term between birth weight and sex reached a p value lower or equal to 0.1, results were reported separately for men and women.

Results are presented as standardized regression coefficients (B), and the statistical significance of the regression coefficient was set at $p = 0.05$.

Results

Descriptive results show that mean birth weight was 3.57 (± 0.51) kg for men and 3.41 (± 0.49) kg for women. Only 7 subjects reported a birth weight lower power or equal to 2.50 kg, which is often considered as low. Characteristics for all other outcome or confounding variables are presented in table 1.

Results from the GEE analyses for the relationships between birth weight and body composition in adulthood are presented in figure 2. As can be seen, no significant associations were observed between birth weight and BMI and FM. In this latter relationship, sex appeared to be an effect modifier (p = 0.1) and therefore, results are presented separately for men and women. Furthermore, in women 'time of measurement' was a significant inverse effect modifier (p = 0.014), but only after adjustment for adult weight. This inverse interaction term indicates that the association between birth weight and FM strengthens with time.

A highly significant positive association (standardized B = 0.121; p < 0.001) was observed between birth weight and adult FFM, which decreased but remained significant (standardized B = 0.040; p = 0.016) after adding adult weight into the model.

Furthermore, a significant strong inverse association was detected between birth weight and AF after adjustment for adult weight (standardized B = 0.265; p = 0.011).

Regarding the associations between birth weight and the cardiovascular health indicators (fig. 3), no significant association was observed between birth weight and SBP. For the association between birth weight and DBP, sex was an effect modifier (p = 0.026). The stratified analyses showed a significant inverse association in women after adjustment for adult weight (standardized B = −0.136; p = 0.043).

Another significant inverse relationship, after adjustment for adult weight, was observed between birth weight and TC (standardized B = −0.118; p = 0.016). For the HDL concentration, no significant association was found; however, the association between birth weight and the ratio between TC and HDL was significant after adjustment for adult weight (standardized B = −0.111; p = 0.011).

Furthermore, time of measurement was a significant (p = 0.036) positive effect modifier in the association between birth weight and HDL, indicating that the association between birth weight and adult HDL loses strength with time. Time of measurement was also an effect modifier in the association between birth weight and the TC:HDL ratio, again it indicates the loss of strength of the relationship between birth weight and TC:HDL ratio, since the interaction term was in a negative direction (β = −0.020) while the regression coefficient for birth weight in this model was positive.

No significant relationship was observed between birth weight and the concentration of triglycerides.

The stratified analyses for the relationship between birth weight and VO_2max showed that the associations were in opposite directions for both

Table 1. Characteristics of the study population for men (M) and women (W) concerning body composition, cardiovascular and musculoskeletal health measured at mean ages of 27, 32/33 and 36 years

	27 years		32/33 years		36 years	
	M	W	M	W	M	W
Body composition	n = 53	n = 77	n = 126	n = 183	n = 121	n = 171
Height, m	1.83 ± 0.06	1.70 ± 0.06	1.84 ± 0.06	1.70 ± 0.06	1.84 ± 0.06	1.71 ± 0.06
Weight, kg	76.6 ± 9.2	64.3 ± 7.8	81.5 ± 9.0	66.2 ± 9.0	84.4 ± 10.7	68.6 ± 10.3
BMI, kg/m^2	22.7 ± 2.2	22.2 ± 2.5	24.1 ± 2.4	22.8 ± 3.0	24.7 ± 2.7	23.4 ± 3.4
Waist circumference, cm	78.9 ± 6.1	68.3 ± 5.7	83.0 ± 6.6	71.0 ± 6.7	85.1 ± 8.1	73.5 ± 9.1
Fat mass, kg	11.4 ± 4.5	16.4 ± 4.9	15.7 ± 4.6	18.8 ± 5.0	17.4 ± 4.8	20.0 ± 5.7
Fat free mass, kg	65.1 ± 6.3	47.6 ± 5.0	65.5 ± 5.8	47.1 ± 4.6	66.7 ± 6.8	48.4 ± 5.3
Cardiovascular health	n = 53	n = 77	n = 125	n = 183	n = 121	n = 171
Systolic blood pressure, mm Hg	137.6 ± 10.1	123.6 ± 9.3	136.2 ± 11.9	124.7 ± 10.2	139.1 ± 14.7	124.9 ± 11.3
Diastolic blood pressure, mm Hg	83.1 ± 9.4	80.3 ± 7.7	86.2 ± 8.2	82.9 ± 8.5	89.9 ± 11.5	82.2 ± 9.1
Total cholesterol (TC), mmol/l	5.01 ± 0.9	5.37 ± 0.9	5.08 ± 0.9	4.92 ± 0.8	5.24 ± 0.93	4.88 ± 0.84
HDL cholesterol, mmol/l	1.18 ± 0.23	1.63 ± 0.36	1.20 ± 0.26	1.59 ± 0.35	1.19 ± 0.27	1.57 ± 0.36
TC:HDL ratio	4.39 ± 1.07	3.42 ± 0.84	4.39 ± 1.17	3.21 ± 0.82	4.61 ± 1.30	3.25 ± 0.92
Triglycerides, mmol/l	1.14 ± 0.45	1.08 ± 0.60	1.28 ± 0.80	0.95 ± 0.39	1.65 ± 1.13	0.98 ± 0.42
Maximum oxygen uptake, ml·min^{-1}·kg$^{-2/3}$	213.1 ± 23.5	161.1 ± 18.9	198.3 ± 26.9	162.4 ± 23.9	194.9 ± 26.9	160.7 ± 24.3
Musculoskeletal health	n = 53	n = 73	n = 124	n = 174	n = 120	n = 162
Lumbar (L2–4) BMC, g						
Norland XR 26[1]	62.5 ± 11.2	52.6 ± 8.3	63.8 ± 13.5	52.7 ± 9.2		
Hologic QDR 2000[1]			65.8 ± 12.4	53.3 ± 7.6	65.3 ± 14.1	54.5 ± 8.8
Lumbar (L2–4) BMD, g/cm^2						
Norland XR 26[1]	1.17 ± 0.17	1.14 ± 0.14	1.17 ± 0.19	1.12 ± 0.15		
Hologic QDR 2000[1]			1.12 ± 0.16	1.07 ± 0.10	1.12 ± 0.17	1.09 ± 0.12
Arm pull, kg/kg body weight	0.90 ± 0.16	0.61 ± 0.06	0.92 ± 0.13	0.64 ± 0.11	0.85 ± 0.13	0.57 ± 0.10
High jump, cm	56.2 ± 7.1	43.1 ± 5.4	55.5 ± 7.6	41.3 ± 5.1	53.0 ± 7.2	38.5 ± 5.6

[1]Two different machines were used during the measurements.

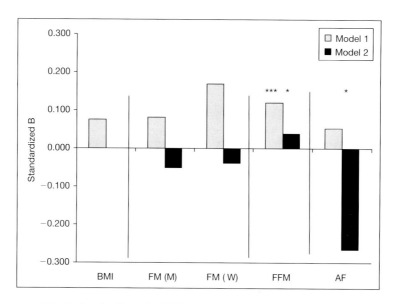

Fig. 2. Results from the GEE analyses for the relationship between birth weight and body composition. FM = Fat mass; FFM = fat-free mass; AF = abdominal fat (waist circumference); M = men; W = women. Model 1 = Adjusted for sex; model 2 = adjusted for sex and adult weight. *p < 0.05, ***p < 0.001.

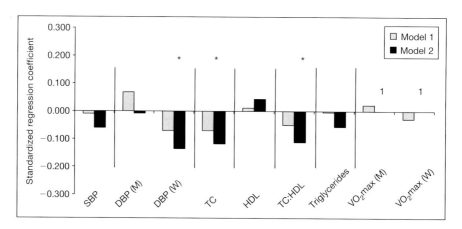

Fig. 3. Results from the GEE analyses for the relationship between birth weight and cardiovascular risk factors. SBP = Systolic blood pressure; DBP = diastolic blood pressure; TC = total cholesterol; HDL = high-density lipoprotein cholesterol; TC:HDL = TC:HDL ratio; M = men; W = women. Model 1 = adjusted for sex; model 2 = adjusted for sex and adult weight (not analyzed for VO₂max)[1]. *p < 0.05; ***p < 0.001.

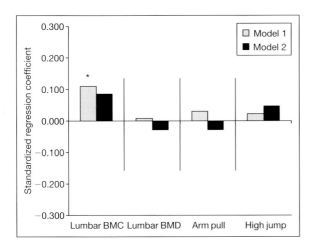

Fig.4. Results from the GEE analyses for the relationship between birth weight and musculoskeletal health. BMC = Bone mineral content; BMD = bone mineral density. Model 1 = adjusted for sex; model 2 = adjusted for sex and adult weight.

sexes (p value for interaction = 0.1), but none of those were statistically significant.

The studied relationships between birth weight and musculoskeletal health indicators showed only one significant association, namely between birth weight and lumbar BMC (standardized B = 0.111; p = 0.031). However, this association decreased slightly after adjustment for adult weight. The results are presented in figure 4.

To analyze whether or not FFM is a mediator in the possible associations between birth weight and cardiovascular and musculoskeletal health, additional analyses were performed. From figure 2, it is clear that birth weight is indeed associated with adult FFM; furthermore, figures 3 and 4 show associations between birth weight and DBP (in women), TC, TC:HDL and lumbar BMC. Besides, in the population of the AGAHLS, FFM is inversely related to DBP, TC and TC:HDL after adjustment for adult weight (p values between 0.015 and 0.077, data not shown), and positively to lumbar BMC [18]. Therefore, additional analyses were performed to study the intermediating effect of FFM in the associations between birth weight and DBP (in women), TC, TC:HDL and lumbar BMC, by adding FFM in a statistical model which already included birth weight, sex and time of measurement. Results showed that the changes in the regression coefficient for birth weight are comparable with the changes in the regression coefficient when adult body weight was included in the model, as can be seen in figure 5.

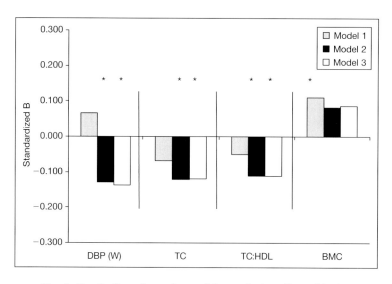

Fig. 5. Results from the analyses of the mediating effect of fat free mass (FFM) in the relationships between birth weight and diastolic blood pressure, total cholesterol (TC), TC:HDL ratio and bone mineral density. DBP = Diastolic blood pressure; TC = total cholesterol; HDL = high-density lipoprotein; BMC = bone mineral content; W = women only; FFM = fat-free mass. Model 1 = Adjusted for sex; model 2 = model + adjusted for FFM; model 3 = model 1 + adjusted for adult weight. *p < 0.05.

Discussion

The aim of the study was to analyze, in the relatively young and apparently healthy population of the AGAHLS, whether birth weight was associated with body composition, cardiovascular and musculoskeletal health, and to study whether FFM had a mediating effect in the associations between birth weight and cardiovascular and musculoskeletal health.

Results showed that birth weight was not associated with BMI or FM, but was indeed associated with FFM which is consistent with others [13–17]. In the AGAHLS population 1 kg increase in birth weight is associated with an increase of 2.5 kg in FFM, which is comparable with what others report. However, the association lost strength, but remained significant, after adding adult weight into the model (0.8 kg increase in FFM for 1 kg higher birth weight).

Furthermore, birth weight was associated with AF, as measured with waist circumference, but only after adjustment for adult weight. Most other studies report on the waist/hip ratio, and not on the waist circumference alone, therefore it is difficult to compare our results with others. Although Ravelli et al. [32]

showed that women who were exposed to famine during early gestation had higher waist circumferences at age 50 years. That those of lower birth weight store their fat more centrally might be explained by an altered hormonal status. It can be that adrenal overactivity is a result from early growth restraint, and also causes a more central fat patterning later in life [33].

Cardiovascular Health

Regarding the cardiovascular health indicators, in this population birth weight seems not to be associated with SBP. However, this might have been caused by the SBP measurement method. Since it was measured with a 5 mm Hg accuracy interval, and from the literature it is known that we can expect an effect of 2–3 mm Hg decrease in SBP with 1 kg increase in birth weight [5]. Besides, it was measured just before the subjects had to start a running test, and this could have caused some stress which in turn can affect SBP. Unpublished data from analyses in the same AGAHLS population show that birth weight is inversely associated with SBP ($\beta = -3.31$, $p = 0.003$) when SBP was accurately measured with an oscillometric device (Colin Press-Mate, model BP-8800, Komaki-City, Japan).

Although the same arguments concerning accuracy do hold for the measurement of DBP, a significant inverse association (after adjustment for adult weight) was found with birth weight, but only in women.

Furthermore, in the present study birth weight was inversely associated with TC and TC:HDL, again only after adjustment for adult weight. The published literature on this issue is limited and conflicting, and therefore it is hard to compare results. One study that addressed this association was a study performed in adults aged between 50 and 53 years [8], and showed inverse non significant trends between birth weight and TC. However, when they used abdominal circumference at birth as a measure of intra-uterine growth, the observed results were statistically significant. Ziegler et al. [34] report an inverse association between birth weight and TC in men, aged between 30 and 50 years. That birth weight is inversely related to TC might be a result of impaired liver growth and subsequent altered cholesterol metabolism.

Another study, also performed in the UK reported that in women low birth weight was associated with lower levels of serum HDL and raised triglycerides concentrations [7], both associations could not be confirmed in our younger population.

Finally, we studied the relationship between birth weight and cardio-pulmonary fitness and observed opposite effects for men and women,; however, neither associations were significant. To the best of our knowledge, this issue was not addressed by others. Only Baraldi et al. [35] report on results from very low birth weight (VLBW) children and exercise performance at ages between

9 and 12 years. They show that these VLBW weight children did not differ from their controls, who were born at term and appropriate for gestational age, on maximum oxygen consumption and anaerobic threshold. These VLBW children were more extreme regarding their birth weights than the subjects assessed in the AGAHLS; therefore, it is not surprising that we did not find significant associations between birth weight and maximum oxygen uptake.

Musculoskeletal Health

In the present study, only one significant association was observed between birth weight and indicators of musculoskeletal health, which was between birth weight and lumbar BMC. This observation is consistent with those reported by others [13, 36]. However, this association decreased after adding adult weight into the model. This is not surprising since BMC is strongly related to body weight, and birth weight is also strongly related to later body weight. That no relationship was observed between birth weight and lumber BMD can therefore be expected, since BMD is already a measure relative for size. In sum, it seems that birth weight is related to bone mass, but not to bone density. It is suggested that the growth hormone (GH) insulin-like growth factor (IGF) axis (GH-IGF-axis) is involved since there are abnormalities in the GH-IGF axis in growth-retarded infants, and altered levels of these hormones are also related to increased risk for osteoporosis [37].

Furthermore, no significant associations were observed between birth weight and muscle strength, as measured with arm pull and high jump. This is in contrast with what others reported [19]. No clear explanations can be given why no associations were detected in this population since lower birth weight was related to lower FFM, which is known to be related to muscle strength.

Mediating Effect of FFM

A second aim of present study was to investigate the mediating effect of FFM in possible relationships between birth weight and cardiovascular on musculoskeletal health. In this study birth weight was indeed positively associated with FFM, even after adjustment for adult weight (fig. 2).

The mediating effect of FFM was studied by adding FFM as a time-dependent co-variate in a statistical model which already included birth weight, sex and time of measurement. As mentioned before, the results were the same as with adjustment for body weight, i.e. changes in the regression coefficient for birth weight were comparable (fig. 5). That the studied relationships become only significant after adjustment for adult body weight or adult FFM can be explained by the fact that birth weight is positively associated with adult body weight and FFM, and that adult body weight and FFM are inversely associated with the studied health indicators. If then the associations are studied in a crude model, the combined result of these positive and negative associations is no association. But, when adjustments are made for either adult body weight or FFM, the inverse association becomes visible. It can therefore be argued that this is a mediating effect, but this mediating effect of FFM is not different from the effect of adjustment for adult weight.

Conclusions

This study shows that in a young and apparently healthy population of the AGAHLS birth weight is significantly positively associated with FFM, and inversely with AF after adjustment for adult weight. Furthermore, birth weight was associated with some indicators for cardiovascular health, namely inversely with DBP (in women only), TC and TC:HDL ratio and positively to only one indicator of musculoskeletal health, lumbar BMC. However, this latter relationship decreased after adding adult weight (or height) into the model.

Since the associations between birth weight and DBP, TC, TC:HDL become stronger after adjustment for FFM and the relationship between birth weight and BMC lost significance after adjustment for FFM, FFM can be seen as a mediator in these relationships.

References

1   Barker DJ: Early growth and cardiovascular disease. Arch Dis Child 1999;80:305–307.
2   Barker DJ: In utero programming of chronic disease. Clin Sci (Lond) 1998;95:115–128.
3   Barker M, Robinson S, Osmond C, Barker DJ: Birth weight and body fat distribution in adolescent girls. Arch Dis Child 1997;77:381–383.
4   Barker DJ: Intrauterine programming of coronary heart disease and stroke. Acta Paediatr Suppl 1997;423:178–82; discussion 183.
5   Law CM, Shiell AW: Is blood pressure inversely related to birth weight? The strength of evidence from a systematic review of the literature. J Hypertens 1996;14:935–941.
6   Barker DJ: The intrauterine origins of cardiovascular disease. Acta Paediatr Suppl 1993; 82(suppl 391):93–9; discussion 100.
7   Fall CH, Osmond C, Barker DJ, Clark PM, Hales CN, Stirling Y, Meade TW: Fetal and infant growth and cardiovascular risk factors in women. BMJ 1995;310:428–432.
8   Barker DJ, Martyn CN, Osmond C, Hales CN, Fall CH: Growth in utero and serum cholesterol concentrations in adult life. BMJ 1993;307:1524–1527.
9   Roseboom TJ, van der Meulen JH, Osmond C, Barker DJ, Ravelli AC, Bleker OP: Plasma lipid profiles in adults after prenatal exposure to the Dutch famine. Am J Clin Nutr 2000;72: 1101–1106.
10 Frankel S, Elwood P, Sweetnam P, Yarnell J, Smith GD: Birth weight, body-mass index in middle age, and incident coronary heart disease. Lancet 1996;348:1478–1480.
11 Rich-Edwards JW, Stampfer MJ, Manson JE, Rosner B, Hankinson SE, Colditz GA, Willett WC, Hennekens CH: Birth weight and risk of cardiovascular disease in a cohort of women followed up since 1976. BMJ 1997;315:396–400.

12 Tenhola S, Martikainen A, Rahiala E, Herrgard E, Halonen P, Voutilainen R: Serum lipid concen-
    trations and growth characteristics in 12-year-old children born small for gestational age. Pediatr
    Res 2000;48:623–628.

13 Gale CR, Martyn CN, Kellingray S, et al: Intrauterine programming of adult body composition.
    J Clin Endocrinol Metab 2001;86,1:267–272.

14 Singhal A, Wells J, Cole TJ, Fewtrell M, Lucas A: Programming of lean body mass: A link between
    birth weight, obesity, and cardiovascular disease? Am J Clin Nutr 2003;77:726–730.

15 Loos RJ, Beunen G, Fagard R, Derom C, Vlietinck R: Birth weight and body composition in
    young adult men: A prospective twin study. Int J Obes Relat Metab Disord 2001;25:1537–1545.

16 Loos RJ, Beunen G, Fagard R, Derom C, Vlietinck R: Birth weight and body composition in
    young women: A prospective twin study. Am J Clin Nutr 2002;75:676–682.

17 Eriksson J, Forsen T, Tuomilehto J, Osmond C, Barker D: Size at birth, fat-free mass and resting
    metabolic rate in adult life. Horm Metab Res 2002;34:72–76.

18 Bakker I, Twisk JWR, van Mechelen W, Kemper HCG: Fat-free body mass is the most important
    body composition determinant of 10-year longitudinal development of lumbar bone in adult men
    and women. J Clin Endocrinol Metab, in press.

19 Kuh D, Bassey J, Hardy R, Aihie Sayer A, Wadsworth M, Cooper C: Birth weight, childhood size,
    and muscle strength in adult life: Evidence from a birth cohort study. Am J Epidemiol 2002;156:
    627–633.

20 Axelsson G, Rylander R: Validation of questionnaire reported miscarriage, malformation and
    birth weight. Int J Epidemiol 1984;13:94–98.

21 Hoekelman RA, Kelly J, Zimmer AW: The reliability of maternal recall. Mother's remembrance of
    their infant's health and illness. Clin Pediatr (Phila) 1976;15:261–265.

22 Little RE: Birthweight and gestational age: Mothers' estimates compared with state and hospital
    records. Am J Publ Hlth 1986;76:1350–1351.

23 Tilley BC, Barnes AB, Bergstralh E, Labarthe D, Noller KL, Colton T, Adam E: A comparison
    of pregnancy history recall and medical records: Implications for retrospective studies. Am J
    Epidemiol 1985;121:269–281.

24 Weiner JS, Lourie J: Human Biology: A Guide to Field Methods. IBP Handbook No 9. Oxford,
    Blackwell, 1968.

25 Durnin JV, Womersley J: Body fat assessed from total body density and its estimation from
    skinfold thickness: Measurements on 481 men and women aged from 16 to 72 years. Br J Nutr
    1974;32:77–97.

26 Taylor RW, Keil D, Gold EJ, Williams SM, Goulding A: Body mass index, waist girth, and
    waist-to-hip ratio as indexes of total and regional adiposity in women: Evaluation using receiver
    operating characteristic curves. Am J Clin Nutr 1998;67:44–49.

27 Huang TC, Chen CP, Wefler V, Raftery A: A stable reagent for the Liberman Buchard reaction:
    Application to rapid serum cholesterol determination. Anal Chem 1961;33:1405–1407.

28 Burnstein M, Samaille J: Sur un dosage rapide du cholesterol lie aux alpha- et aux betalipopro-
    teines du serum. Clin Chim Acta 1960;5:609–611.

29 Kemper HCG, Verschuur R: Maximal aerobic power in 13- and 14-year-old teenagers in relation
    to biologic age. Int J Sports Med 1981;2:97–100.

30 Kemper HCG: The Amsterdam Growth Study: A Longitudinal Analyses of Health, Fitness and
    Lifestyle. HK Sport Science Monograph Series, No 6. Champaign, Human Kinetics, 1995.

31 Diggle JP, Liang KY, Zeger S L: Analyses of Longitudinal Data, ed 1. Oxford, Oxford University
    Press, 2000.

32 Ravelli AC, van Der Meulen JH, Osmond C, Barker DJ, Bleker OP: Obesity at the age of 50 y in
    men and women exposed to famine prenatally. Am J Clin Nutr 1999;70:811–816.

33 Byrne CD, Phillips DI: Fetal origins of adult disease: Epidemiology and mechanisms. J Clin
    Pathol 2000;53:822–828.

34 Ziegler B, Johnsen SP, Thulstrup AM, Engberg M, Lauritzen T, Sorensen HT: Inverse association
    between birth weight, birth length and serum total cholesterol in adulthood. Scand Cardiovasc J
    2000;34:584–588.

35 Baraldi E, Zanconato S, Zorzi C, Santuz P, Benini F, Zacchello F: Exercise performance in very
    low birth weight children at the age of 7–12 years. Eur J Pediatr 1991;150:713–716.

36   Yarbrough DE, Barrett-Connor E, Morton DJ: Birth weight as a predictor of adult bone mass in postmenopausal women: The Rancho Bernardo Study. Osteoporos Int 2000;11:626–630.
37   Holt RI: Fetal programming of the growth hormone-insulin-like growth factor axis. Trends Endocrinol Metab 2002;13:392–397.

Prof. Dr. Han C.G. Kemper
AGAHLS Research Group, Institute for Research in Extramural Medicine
VU University Medical Center
Van der Boechorststraat 7, NL–1081 BT Amsterdam (The Netherlands)
Tel. +31 20 4448407, Fax +31 20 4446775, E-Mail hcg.kemper.emgo@med.vu.nl

Kemper HCG (ed): Amsterdam Growth and Health Longitudinal Study.
Med Sport Sci. Basel, Karger, 2004, vol 47, pp 78–100

....

Fitness and Fatness in Adolescence and Adulthood as Determinants of Large Artery Properties at Age 36

Isabel Ferreira[a], *Jos W.R. Twisk*[a,b], *Willem van Mechelen*[a,c],
Coen D.A. Stehouwer[a,d], *Han C.G. Kemper*[a]

[a]Institute for Research in Extramural Medicine, [b]Department of Clinical
Epidemiology and Biostatistics, [c]Department of Social Medicine and
Body@Work, Research Centre for Physical Activity, Work and Health TNO-VU, and
[d]Department of Internal Medicine and the Institute for Cardiovascular Research,
VU University Medical Center, Amsterdam, The Netherlands

Abstract

Background/Aims: Low levels of cardiorespiratory fitness (VO_2max), and excess total and central fatness are associated with increased cardiovascular risk, but little is known to what extent this is related to their effects on atherosclerosis and arterial stiffness. Moreover, the time-course of these relationships and the relative effects of fitness and total and central fatness need to be elucidated. We therefore investigated the relationships between fitness, total and central fatness on the one hand (determinants) and large-artery properties on the other (outcomes). This was done cross-sectionally (at age 36) and prospectively (i.e. determinants measured during adolescence and outcomes at age 36). *Methods:* Arterial properties were assessed non-invasively by ultrasound imaging. VO_2max was measured with a maximal running test on a treadmill. Total and central fatness were assessed by anthropometry. Cross-sectional analyses consisted of 345 subjects (180 women) and prospective analyses of a sub-population of 159 subjects (84 girls). *Results:* Current and adolescent levels of fitness were inversely and independently associated with carotid IMT, a pre-clinical indicator of atherosclerosis, but only in men. Total and central fatness (the latter in men only) during adolescence, but not at age 36, were positively and independently associated with carotid IMT. Only current levels of fitness were positively associated with arterial stiffness. Central but not overall fatness was independently associated with arterial stiffness and some of these associations had their roots already in adolescence. There were no significant fitness-fatness/central fatness interactions in the above relationships. *Conclusion:* Both low levels of fitness and high levels of fatness, in particular central fatness, can be deleterious for large-artery properties, independently of each other and other risk factors. As the roots of these associations were already present in adolescence this study supports public health policies aiming at the improvement of fitness and decrease of (central) fatness starting early in life.

Atherosclerosis and increased arterial stiffness are causes of cardiovascular disease [1, 2], the former by increasing the risk of atherothrombotic events [3], and the latter by its contribution to systolic hypertension, left ventricular hypertrophy and impaired coronary perfusion [4–7]. The development of non-invasive ultrasound imaging techniques in the last decade has allowed the investigation of such structural and functional changes in large arteries. Ultrasound-assessed carotid intima media thickness (IMT) is thus extensively used as a marker of the atherosclerotic burden [8], and arterial stiffness is most often expressed in terms of distensibility, compliance, elastic modulus and pulse wave velocity [2].

High levels of cardiorespiratory fitness are associated with reduced cardiovascular disease [9–11], and this can be due, at least partially, to the beneficial impact of fitness on carotid IMT [12–14], at least in men, and on arterial stiffness [12, 15–17]. Body fatness [18–21], and in particular a central pattern of fat distribution [22, 23], has also been associated with increased cardiovascular risk. Total [24–28] and central fatness [24, 26, 28–30] are related to higher carotid IMT. Associations of total and/or central fatness with arterial stiffness have shown contradictory results [31–35], but this might be due to the different associations of diverse estimates of total and central fatness (i.e. different fat depots) and estimates of stiffness at different sites in the arterial tree (e.g. elastic vs. muscular arteries) [36]. Moreover, the associations between obesity on the one hand, and atherosclerosis and arterial stiffness on the other, may originate quite early in life [18, 37–40]. However, the impact of central fatness during adolescence on adult atherosclerosis and arterial stiffness is not known, and studies on the association of adolescent fitness with the same adult outcomes are scarce [12]. Understanding the earliest determinants of arterial impairment can have important implications for public health policies targeting young people. An aspect that also needs to be addressed is that these two important cardiovascular risk factors, fitness and (central) fatness, are inversely related [41, 42], and therefore their associations with atherosclerosis and arterial stiffness, independently of each other, need to be clarified.

A further question of great public health importance is whether fitness can reduce the adverse impact of fatness on cardiovascular risk. This has been suggested by studies on an extensive cohort of men [43–45], but recently not corroborated in another extensive cohort of both men and women [46]. Fitness-fatness or fitness-central fatness interactions with regard to their associations with atherosclerosis and arterial stiffness have not yet been addressed. Any such interactions can provide important information on the value of strategies to improve physical fitness in specific populations as a means to prevent adverse cardiovascular outcomes.

In the Amsterdam Growth and Health Longitudinal Study (AGAHLS), measures of cardiopulmonary fitness, total and central fatness gathered from adolescence into adulthood [36, 47], and the assessment of carotid IMT and arterial stiffness estimates gathered at age 36 [12, 36], provide an opportunity to study these issues. Therefore, the purpose of the present study was 3-fold: (1) to examine the independent associations of fitness and total and central fatness on the one hand, and carotid IMT and stiffness at different sites of the arterial tree (i.e. at the elastic carotid and the muscular femoral arteries) on the other (cross-sectional analyses at age 36); (2) to investigate the independent associations of fitness and total and central fatness during adolescence (13–16 years) and these arterial properties at the age of 36 years (prospective analyses), and (3) to investigate the combined effects of fitness and total/central fatness on the above associations, i.e. in both the cross-sectional and the prospective approaches.

Methods

Subjects and Study Design

The AGAHLS is an observational longitudinal study that started in 1977 with a group of 450 boys and girls. Its initial goal was to describe the natural development of growth, health and lifestyle of adolescents, and to investigate longitudinal relationships between biological and lifestyle variables. The mean age of the subjects at the beginning of the study was 13.1 ($\pm$0.8) years. Since then, subjects have been measured 2–8 times during a 24-year follow-up period. At each measurement, anthropometrical (body height, weight and skinfolds), biological (serum lipoprotein levels, blood pressure and physical fitness), lifestyle (nutrient intake, smoking behavior, daily physical activity) and psychological variables were assessed. In the most recent measurement period (in 2000), when the subjects' mean age was 36.5 ($\pm$0.6) years, large artery properties as assessed by non-invasive ultrasound imaging were investigated for the first time. Analyses reported herein include 165 men and 180 women (cross-sectional analyses at age 36), as well as subjects who had had at least 3 of the 4 possible fitness and anthropometric measurements during adolescence (13–16 years) and subsequent evaluations of these variables at age 36 – a subpopulation of 75 men and 84 women (prospective analyses) (fig. 1). The study was approved by the medical ethical committee of the VU University Medical Center, Amsterdam, The Netherlands, and all subjects gave their written informed consent (provided by the parents when the subjects were 13–16 years of age).

Cardiorespiratory Fitness

Throughout the years cardiorespiratory fitness was measured in the same laboratory with the same protocol and equipment: a maximal running test on a treadmill (Quinton 18–54, USA) with direct measurements of oxygen uptake – VO_2max (Ergoanalyzer, Jaeger, The Netherlands). Subjects were instructed to run at a constant speed of 8 km/h while the slope of the treadmill increased every 2 min in a stepwise fashion, and were encouraged to keep running to their maximum. A detailed description of this measurement is given elsewhere [48]. VO_2max was used as a measure of fitness and its values scaled to body size (i.e.

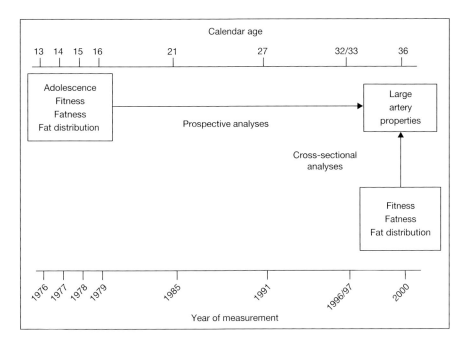

Fig. 1. Study design.

in $ml \cdot min^{-1} \cdot kg^{-2/3}$) were used in the analyses. This allometric scale approach was used due to the high dependency of VO_2max on body size during growth [49].

Anthropometry

Standing height was measured with a Harpenden digital readout, wall-mounted or portable stadiometer (Holtain, UK: van Rietschoten and Houwens, The Netherlands). Body weight was measured with a spring balance (Van Vucht, The Netherlands). The biceps, triceps, subscapular and suprailiac skinfolds were measured to the nearest millimeter with a Harpenden calliper (Holtain, UK). The sum of these four skinfolds (S4S) was used as an indicator of total fatness. The ratio between the subscapular + suprailiac and the ΣSKF (SKF ratio) was used as an estimate of central (subcutaneous) fatness [47]. Throughout the years, all the anthropometric measurements were performed by trained observers according to the guidelines of the International Biological Program [50].

Arterial Properties

All subjects had abstained from smoking and caffeine-containing beverages on the day the measurements were performed. At the time of measurements of arterial properties, subjects had been resting in a supine position for 15 min in a quiet, temperature-controlled room.

Properties of the right common carotid, the common femoral and the brachial arteries were obtained by two trained vascular sonographers with the use of an ultrasound scanner equipped with a 7.5-MHz linear array probe (Pie Medical, Maastricht, The Netherlands). The ultrasound scanner was connected to a personal computer equipped with an acquisition

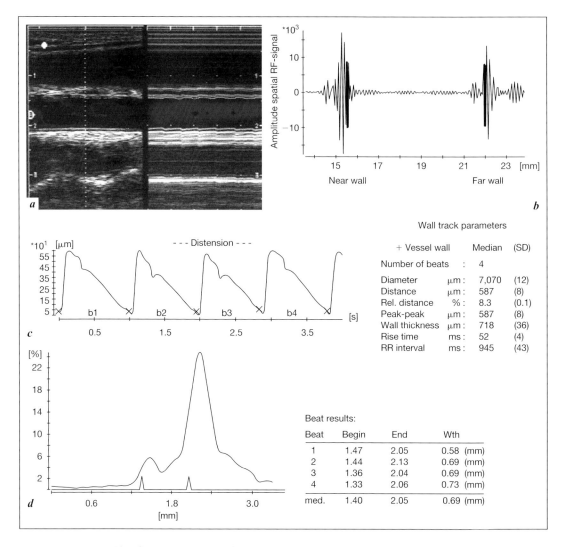

Fig. 2. a B + M-mode image of a common carotid artery in a normal subject. *b* Corresponding radio frequency (RF) signal with automated identification of near and far walls. *c* Artery distension curves over 4s (4 cardiac cycles). *d* Automated measure of carotid IMT based on the RF signal of the posterior wall.

system and a vessel wall movement detector software system (Wall Track System 2, Pie Medical) (WTS2). This integrated device enables measurements of arterial diameter, distension and IMT as described in detail elsewhere [51–53]. Briefly, the artery of interest was visualised in B-mode. An M-line perpendicular to the artery was then placed at the site of measurements. After switching to B + M-mode (fig. 2a), data acquisition was enabled after identification of the lumen of the artery (with the mouse) in a real-time A-mode presentation on the computer screen. Ultrasound data were then obtained during a period of 4 s (including 3–7 heartbeats) triggered by the R-top of the simultaneously recorded ECG. The first radiofrequency (RF) signal was displayed on the screen, enabling the observer to check if the markers, automatically positioned by the WTS2, coincided with the near (adventitia-media) and far (media-adventitia) vessel wall reflections in the diastolic phase of the cardiac cycle (fig. 2b). The cumulative RF signals were then digitized and stored in the computer memory. Diastolic diameter (D) was calculated as the difference in position between the anterior and posterior vessels wall markers and the change in diameter as a function of time (distension [ΔD]) was estimated and presented on the computer screen (distension waveform – fig. 2c). Based on the RF signals of the carotid posterior wall, the distance from the leading edge interface between lumen and intima to the leading edge interface between media and adventitia was calculated automatically as the intima-media complex (fig. 2d). The mean diameter, distension and, for the carotid artery only, IMT, of three consecutive measurements were used in the analyses. The carotid artery was measured approximately 10 mm proximal to the beginning of the bulb, the femoral artery 20 mm proximal to the flow divider and the brachial artery approximately 20 mm above the antecubital fossa. Inter-observer coefficients of variation for the measurements studied on the present report were: carotid intima-media thickness, 11.0%; diameter, 2.9% (carotid) and 2.8% (femoral); and distension, 6.4% (carotid) and 24.2% (femoral). Throughout the entire period of ultrasound imaging, systolic, diastolic and mean arterial pressure (MAP) were assessed in the left arm at 5-min intervals with an oscillometric device (Colin Press-Mate, model BP-8800, Komaki-City, Japan). Brachial artery pulse pressure was defined as systolic minus diastolic blood pressure, and pulse pressure at the common carotid and femoral arteries (i.e. the target arteries) was calculated by calibration of the distension waveforms (using the brachial artery as the reference artery) [54].

Arterial Distensibility, Compliance and Young's Elastic Modulus
Diameter and distension as described above, and the mean local pulse pressure (ΔP) of three measurements obtained at approximately the same time, were used to estimate the distensibility (DC) and compliance (CC) coefficients as follows [53]:

$$DC = \frac{(2\Delta D \cdot D + \Delta D^2)}{(\Delta P \cdot D^2)} \qquad \text{in } 10^{-3} \cdot kPa^{-1} \qquad (1)$$

$$CC = \Pi \cdot \frac{(2D \cdot \Delta D + \Delta D^2)}{4\Delta P} \qquad \text{in } mm^2 \cdot kPa^{-1} \qquad (2)$$

Distensibility reflects the elastic properties whereas compliance reflects the buffering capacity of the artery. From the IMT, diameter and distensibility coefficient of the carotid artery, we calculated Young's elastic modulus (E_{inc}), an estimate of the intrinsic elastic properties of the vessel wall [52]:

$$E_{inc} = \frac{D}{(IMT \cdot DC)} \qquad \text{in } kPa \qquad (3)$$

Lifestyle Risk Factors

Daily physical activity was measured by a structured interview [48]. In this interview, the intensity, frequency and duration of all physical activities (at school, at work, at home, in organized and unorganized sport activities, during leisure time, climbing stairs and transportation) covering the past three months were measured. The time spent on the different activities was then combined with the intensity of the activities to calculate a total weighted activity score (expressed in metabolic equivalents – METs/week). Dietary intake was measured by a detailed cross-check dietary interview, which was specially tailored for use in the AGAHLS [55]. All subjects were asked to recall their usual dietary intake by reporting frequency, amounts and methods of preparation of the foods consumed during the previous month. All consumed food items were then transformed into nutrients according to the Dutch Food Composition Table. The daily intake of the following nutrients were considered in the present study: (1) the intake of fat (expressed as % of total energy intake); (2) the intake of carbohydrates (expressed as % of total energy intake); and the Keys score, which combines the intake of saturated and polyunsaturated fatty acids (both expressed as % of total energy intake), and the intake of cholesterol (in mg/1,000 kcal) [56]. With the dietary history interview, alcohol consumption (in g/week) was also assessed. Smoking status (yes/no) was assessed by a separate questionnaire.

Biological Risk Factors

Total and HDL cholesterol were measured from blood samples (10 ml) taken in the antecubital vein. Standard methods were used and external quality control took place with target samples from a World Health Organisation reference laboratory (Lipid Standardization Laboratory, Atlanta, Ga., USA). After the subjects had been sitting on a chair for 5 min, systolic and diastolic (phase V) blood pressure were measured twice with a sphygmomanometer (Speidell-Keller, Franken & Itallie, The Netherlands) and the lower values were recorded (in mm Hg). Resting heart rate (mean from 15 R-R intervals in the last 15 s of the minute) was measured telemetrically (Telecust 36 and Sirecust BS1, Siemens, The Netherlands). During adolescence, biological age was determined by measuring skeletal age from X-ray photographs of the left hand according to the Tanner-Whitehouse II method, and was used as an indicator of biological maturation.

Statistical Analysis

Mean values ($\pm$ SD) of VO_2max, ΣSKF and the SKR ratio, and of each covariate, were calculated over the adolescent age period for the subjects that met the inclusion criteria. Arterial properties, and estimates of fitness and total and central fatness at age 36 did not differ between subjects excluded and those included in the prospective analyses (data not shown). We then used multiple linear regression analyses to investigate the relationships between fitness, total and central fatness on the one hand (determinants), and arterial properties (outcome variables) on the other. All relationships were analyzed in four steps: firstly, with adjustment for gender, biological age, current height and MAP as measured by the oscillometric device, the latter for arterial stiffness variables only (model 1); secondly, the lifestyle variables were included in the model, since these variables could confound these relationships (model 2); thirdly, we added estimates of total or central fatness or fitness to the previous model in order to assess the (in)dependency of the associations from these variables (model 3), and, fourthly, this model was further adjusted for other biological risk factors that could be both confounders and/or intermediate variables in the associations investigated (model 4). After we had assessed the main effects, we added interaction terms between the determinants and gender to the regression models. When the p value of the interaction terms was <0.1 in the cross-sectional analyses and <0.15 in the prospective analyses, stratified analyses were performed. To facilitate direct comparisons, results of these regression analyses were standardized. A standardized regression coefficient of 0.1 indicates that when the independent variable differed 1 SD between subjects, the dependent differed by 0.1 SD.

To address the eventual protective effect of fitness in 'fat' or 'centrally fat' individuals, we divided the subjects into 4 categories: fit-not fat (or not centrally fat), the reference group; fit-fat; unfit-fat; and unfit-not fat, and investigated if arterial properties differed between these groups. For these analyses, subjects were first categorized as fit/unfit, fat/not fat or centrally fat/not centrally fat by using the highest gender-specific tertile of VO_2max, ΣSKF and the SKR ratio vs. the other tertiles.

All analyses were carried out with the Statistical Package of Social Sciences, 10.1 for Windows (SPSS, Inc., Chicago, Ill., USA). The level of significance was set at $p < 0.05$.

Results

Table 1 shows the mean values of fitness, total and central fatness variables and all covariates considered in the present study, for the cross-sectional and the prospective analyses. Table 2 shows data on large artery properties at the age of 36.

Cross-Sectional Analyses (table 3)

Carotid IMT. VO_2max was inversely associated with carotid IMT in men only. This inverse association was independent of lifestyle, total and central fatness and other biological risk factors. The ΣSKF and the SKF ratio were not associated with carotid IMT.

Arterial Stiffness. In crude and adjusted analyses, VO_2max was positively and significantly associated with carotid distensibility and with the compliance of both the carotid and the femoral arteries. Only after adjustment for biological risk factors other than total or central fatness (i.e. model 4) did the strength of these associations decrease slightly. This was mainly due to adjustments for resting heart rate. The ΣSKF was inversely associated with the compliance of the femoral artery, but these associations weakened considerably after adjustment for fitness, and were then no longer significant. The SKF ratio was positively and significantly associated with Young's elastic modulus, and inversely with distensibility of the carotid artery. After adjustment for other biological risk factors these associations weakened and were no longer significant. This was mainly due to adjustments for cholesterol levels. The SKF ratio was also inversely associated with the compliance of the femoral artery, in men only. Adjustment for fitness weakened this association, although it remained statistically significant.

Table 1. Characteristics of the study population

	Age 36		Adolescence	
	men (n = 165)	women (n = 180)	boys (n = 75)	girls (n = 84)
Fitness				
VO_2max, ml·min·kg$^{-2/3}$	222.3 ± 29.8	166.4 ± 22.5	223.9 ± 16.5	182.7 ± 12.8
Fatness/fat distribution				
S4S, mm	47.0 ± 15.5	55.2 ± 19.7	27.6 ± 8.2	41.6 ± 14.3
SKF ratio	0.65 ± 0.05	0.50 ± 0.07	0.53 ± 0.05	0.51 ± 0.05
Lifestyle covariates				
Daily physical activity, 10^3 METs/week	3.9 (2.1–5.8)	4.5 (3.0–6.7)	4.0 (3.0–4.0)	3.3 (2.7–4.1)
Fat intake, %	33.5 ± 5.5	33.6 ± 4.7	40.0 ± 3.9	38.4 ± 3.7
Carbohydrates intake, %	45.0 ± 6.4	45.7 ± 6.2	46.6 ± 3.8	47.4 ± 3.6
Keys score	41.2 ± 8.2	42.6 ± 8.5	53.6 ± 7.6	51.6 ± 7.5
Alcohol consumption, g/week	94.4 (30.1–184.5)	45.0 (3.2–102.1)	0.4 (0.0–10.0)	1.8 (0.0–9.6)
Smokers, %	27.9	18.9	16.0	29.8
Biological covariates				
Biological age	–	–	14.7 ± 0.9	14.2 ± 1.0
Body height, cm	183.7 ± 6.4	170.3 ± 6.4	–	–
Sitting height, cm	93.5 ± 7.4	87.5 ± 3.3	–	–
Mean arterial pressure, mm Hg*	85.6 ± 7.6	79.0 ± 8.2	–	–
Systolic pressure, mm Hg	138.6 ± 14.0	124.8 ± 11.2	127.4 ± 7.3	122.4 ± 8.1
Diastolic pressure, mm Hg	89.0 ± 10.9	82.3 ± 9.2	73.0 ± 6.3	76.0 ± 5.7
Total cholesterol, mmol/l	5.17 ± 1.00	4.81 ± 0.79	4.18 ± 0.59	4.37 ± 0.63
HDL cholesterol, mmol/l	1.22 ± 0.28	1.57 ± 0.33	1.35 ± 0.20	1.38 ± 0.24
Total/HDL cholesterol	4.48 ± 1.34	3.20 ± 0.92	3.19 ± 0.61	3.27 ± 0.69
Resting heart rate, bpm	68.6 ± 10.4	73.4 ± 10.7	76.1 ± 11.5	82.4 ± 11.3

Data are means ± SD or medians (interquartile range). *As measured by the oscillometric device.

Prospective Analyses (table 4)

Carotid IMT. VO_2max in adolescence was inversely associated with carotid IMT at age 36 in men only. Adjustment for covariates resulted in stronger associations. ΣSKF during adolescence was positively and significantly associated with carotid IMT at age 36 in both crude and adjusted analyses. The SKF ratio was also inversely associated with carotid IMT at age 36 but in men only.

Arterial Stiffness. VO_2max during adolescence was not significantly associated with carotid and femoral arteries distensibility and compliance coefficients. The only relevant association that could be observed was between

Table 2. Large artery properties at the age of 36

	Men (n = 165)	Women (n = 180)
Carotid artery		
Intima-media thickness, mm	0.62 ± 0.10	0.63 ± 0.10
Diameter, mm	7.19 ± 0.51	6.59 ± 0.52
Distension, μm	631 ± 138	517 ± 120
Pulse Pressure, mm Hg	52.8 ± 8.0	45.7 ± 7.8
Distensibility coefficient, $10^{-3} \cdot kPa^{-1}$	26.3 ± 5.3	27.4 ± 6.8
Compliance coefficient, $mm^2 \cdot kPa^{-1}$	1.07 ± 0.27	0.94 ± 0.26
Elastic modulus, $10^3 \cdot kPa$	0.47 ± 0.12	0.42 ± 0.12
Femoral artery		
Diameter, mm	10.58 ± 1.03	8.94 ± 1.07
Distension, μm	222 ± 105	229 ± 96
Pulse pressure, mm Hg	54.1 ± 9.0	49.4 ± 9.9
Distensibility coefficient, $10^{-3} \cdot kPa^{-1}$	6.01 ± 3.06	8.30 ± 4.06
Compliance coefficient, $mm^2 \cdot kPa^{-1}$	0.52 ± 0.25	0.51 ± 0.23

Data are means ± SD.

VO_2max and femoral diameter (data not shown). The SKF ratio during adolescence was inversely associated with the elastic carotid, but not the muscular femoral distensibility and compliance. These associations were independent of fitness and the covariates considered.

Fitness and Fatness Interactions

Figure 3 depicts the percentage of individuals in each fitness-fatness category. In the cross-sectional analyses 24 (21%) and 34 (30%) subjects in the most fit category were fat and centrally fat, respectively (fig. 3a). The corresponding values in prospective analyses were 9 (17%) and 16 (30%) (fig. 3b).

We have then investigated if arterial properties differ between fit-not fat (or not centrally fat), the reference group, fit-fat, unfit-fat and unfit-not fat subjects. This was done in respect to the arterial properties to which either fitness or total or central fatness were independently associated (analyses shown previously).

Carotid IMT. In cross-sectional analyses, there were no interactions between fitness and total and central fatness in the relationships with carotid IMT (fig. 4a, b). However, subjects that were unfit and fat during adolescence had significantly higher carotid IMT at age 36 as compared to the fit-not fat

Table 3. Relationships between fitness, fatness and central fat and large artery properties at age 36

Arterial properties		Fitness – VO$_2$max				Fatness – ΣSKF				Central Fat – SKF ratio			
		model 1	model 2	model 3	model 4	model 1	model 2	model 3	model 4	model 1	model 2	model 3	model 4
Carotid artery													
Intima-media thickness	♂	**–0.21†**	**–0.23†**	**–0.27†/–0.25†**	**–0.21*/–0.20***	0.08	0.09	0.06	0.03	0.05	0.01	0.02	–0.02
	♀	0.04	0.04	0.08/0.04	0.01/–0.00								
Distensibility		**0.18***	**0.19***	**0.19*/0.18***	**0.17*/0.15**	–0.07	–0.06	–0.01	0.02	**–0.18***	**–0.17***	**–0.15***	–0.12
Compliance		**0.20***	**0.21†**	**0.25†/0.20†**	**0.20*/0.17***	–0.03	–0.01	0.06	0.08	–0.06	–0.05	–0.03	–0.02
Elastic modulus		–0.05	–0.06	–0.03/–0.04	–0.05/–0.05	0.05	0.05	0.04	0.01	**0.16***	**0.15**	**0.15**	0.11
Femoral artery													
Distensibility		0.03	0.04	–0.02/0.03	–0.02/0.02	**–0.09**	**–0.10**	**–0.10**	**–0.09**	**–0.15**	**–0.15**	**–0.15**	–0.13
Compliance	♂	**0.27‡**	**0.27‡**	**0.23*/0.25‡**	**0.20*/0.22***	**–0.13***	**–0.12***	–0.06	–0.05	**–0.25†**	**–0.24†**	**–0.19***	**–0.21***
	♀									–0.04	–0.02	–0.02	0.01

Data are standardized regression coefficients.

Model 1: Adjusted for gender, current height and MAP, the latter for arterial stiffness parameters only. Model 2: Further adjusted for lifestyle variables: daily physical activity, fat and carbohydrate intake, Keys score, smoking status and alcohol consumption. Model 3: Further adjusted for ΣSKF or (/) SKF ratio (in analyses with VO$_2$max as the main determinant) or VO$_2$max (in analyses with ΣSKF and SKF ratio as the main determinants). Model 4: Further adjusted for other biological risk factors: ratio total/HDL cholesterol and resting heart rate, and systolic and diastolic blood pressure, the latter in analyses with IMT only. *p < 0.05, † p < 0.01, ‡ p < 0.001; associations with p values <0.1 are in **bold**.

Table 4. Relationships between fitness, fatness and central fat during adolescence and large artery properties at age 36

Arterial properties		Fitness – VO_2max				Fatness – S4S				Central fat-SKF ratio			
		model 1	model 2	model 3	model 4	model 1	model 2	model 3	model 4	model 1	model 2	model 3	model 4
Carotid artery													
Intima-media thickness	♂	**−0.28***	**−0.32***	**−0.30*/−0.28***	**−0.33*/−0.37***	**0.29***	**0.32†**	**0.30†**	**0.28***	**0.23**	**0.24**	**0.26***	**0.26***
	♀	0.07	0.06	0.14/0.06	0.11/−0.01					0.01	0.00	0.00	−0.01
Distensibility		0.09	0.14	0.15/0.15	0.13/0.12	−0.02	0.01	0.03	0.03	**−0.13**	**−0.14**	**−0.14**	**−0.15**
Compliance	♂	−0.07	−0.02	0.03/−0.01	−0.02/−0.07	0.07	0.09	0.11	0.15	**−0.19***	**−0.19***	**−0.19***	**−0.19***
	♀	0.14	0.16	0.17/0.17	0.19/0.16								
Elastic modulus	♂	0.14	0.15	0.12/0.16	0.13/0.17	−0.09	−0.13	−0.14	−0.11	−0.02	−0.01	−0.01	−0.00
	♀	−0.15	−0.18	−0.21/−0.18	−0.22/−0.19								
Femoral artery													
Distensibility		−0.20	−0.18	−0.19/−0.18	−0.20/−0.19	−0.02	−0.01	−0.02	−0.04	0.05	0.02	0.02	0.02
Compliance		−0.08	−0.04	−0.05/−0.04	−0.07/−0.05	−0.01	−0.01	−0.02	−0.04	0.05	0.02	0.02	0.02

Data are standardized regression coefficients.

Model 1: Adjusted for gender, biological age, current height and MAP, the latter for arterial stiffness parameters only. Model 2: Further adjusted for lifestyle variables during adolescence: daily physical activity, fat and carbohydrate intake, Keys score, smoking status and alcohol consumption. Model 3: Further adjusted for adolescent ΣSKF or (/) SKF ratio (in analyses with VO_2max as the main determinant) or adolescent VO_2max (in analyses with ΣSKF and SKF ratio as the main determinants). Model 4: Further adjusted for other biological risk factors during adolescence: ratio total/HDL cholesterol and resting heart rate, and systolic and diastolic blood pressure, the latter in analyses with IMT only. *p < 0.05., †p < 0.01; associations with p values <0.1 are in **bold**.

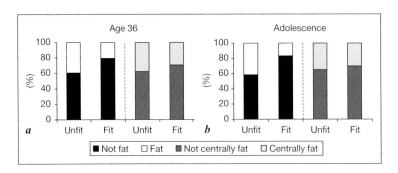

Fig. 3. Percentage of participants classified as 'fat' and 'centrally fat' within fitness categories: (*a*) cross-sectional analyses; (*b*) prospective analyses.

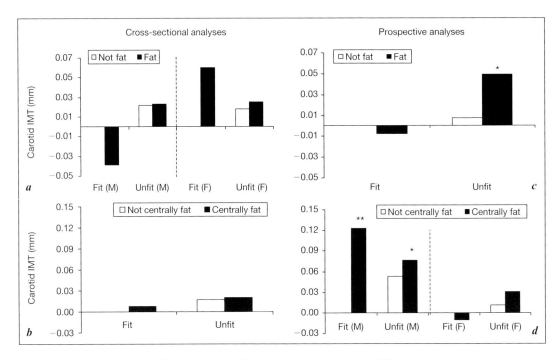

Fig. 4. Differences in carotid IMT between categories of fitness and (*a*) total fatness, (*b*) central fatness, in cross-sectional analyses; (*c*) total fatness, (*d*) central fatness, in prospective analyses; **$p < 0.01$; *$p < 0.05$; †$p < 0.1$. Data are presented separately for men (M) and women (F) when significant interactions with gender were found.

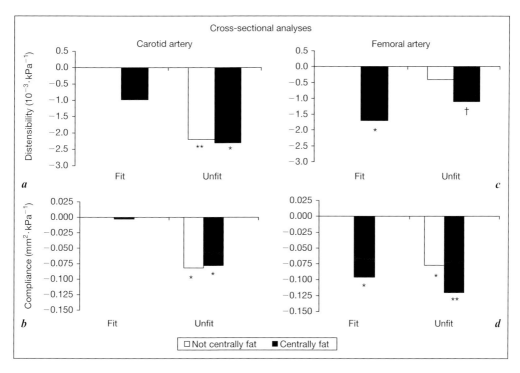

Fig. 5. Differences in stiffness estimates between categories of fitness and central fatness in cross-sectional analyses: (**a**) carotid distensibility; (**b**) carotid compliance; (**c**) femoral distensibility and (**d**) femoral compliance. **p < 0.01, *p < 0.05; †p < 0.1.

subjects. Moreover, fat but fit individuals had comparable carotid IMT to unfit-not fat individuals, but the number of subjects in the former category was very low (n = 9) (fig. 4c). This pattern of differences between groups was not replicated when fitness-central fatness interactions were investigated. In this case, centrally fat boys had significantly higher carotid IMT at age 36 than the fit-not centrally fat boys, independently of their fitness levels (fig. 4d).

Arterial Stiffness. In cross-sectional and prospective analyses, there were no significant fitness-fatness or fitness-central fatness interactions in the relationships with estimates of arterial stiffness. This is illustrated in figures 5 and 6, where the fitness-central fatness combinations are investigated. Unfit subjects, whether centrally fat or not, had significantly lower distensibility and compliance of the carotid artery, while fit but centrally fat individuals had comparable values to the fit-not centrally fat subjects (fig. 5a, b). However, as far as the femoral artery was concerned, centrally fat subjects had lower distensibility and compliance than the fit-not centrally fat (fig. 5c, d). Unfit-not centrally fat also had

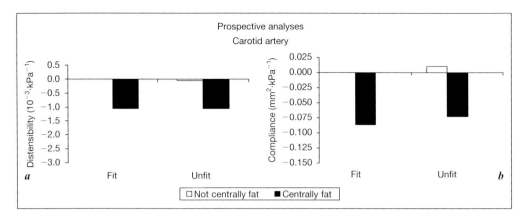

Fig. 6. Differences in stiffness estimates between categories of fitness and central fatness in prospective analyses: (*a*) carotid distensibility; (*b*) carotid compliance.

reduced compliance. In prospective analyses, centrally fat subjects, either fit or unfit, tended to have lower carotid distensibility and compliance, while unfit-not centrally fat individuals had values comparable to those of the reference group. However, none of these associations were statistically significant which might be due to the lower sample size in the prospective analyses (e.g. the magnitude of the differences between groups in carotid compliance was comparable to that of the cross-sectional analyses).

Discussion

The main findings of our study were that: (i) not only current but also adolescent levels of fitness were inversely associated with carotid IMT, a preclinical indicator of atherosclerosis, but only in men; (ii) fatness and truncal subcutaneous fat accumulation (the latter in men only) during adolescence but not at age 36 were positively associated with carotid IMT at age 36; (iii) only current levels of fitness were positively associated with the compliance of both the elastic carotid and the muscular femoral artery, and with carotid but not femoral arterial distensibility; (iv) truncal subcutaneous fat, but not overall fatness, was associated with arterial stiffness and some of these associations had their roots already in adolescence; (v) all the previous associations were independent of fitness or total and central fatness levels and other risk factors, and (vi) overall it did not appear that being fit entirely attenuated the deleterious effects of being fat.

Cardiopulmonary Fitness and Carotid IMT and Arterial Stiffness

Inverse associations between VO_2max and carotid IMT in men are consistent with other studies [13, 14, 57] but not all [58–60]. These discrepancies may reflect differences in the determination of fitness levels (methods and accuracy). Additionally, it can reflect different adaptations to different types of exercise because morphological changes in peripheral vessels have recently been shown to differ among athletes engaged in different types of sports (i.e. greater relative wall thickness in strength-trained than in endurance-trained athletes) [61, 62]. In the present study the association, in men, between VO_2max levels during adolescence and carotid IMT at age 36 suggests that cardiopulmonary fitness at an early age can influence carotid wall thickening much later. This observation was independent of other risk factors, suggesting the existence of a direct link between fitness and arterial thickness. In women, VO_2max was not significantly associated with carotid IMT, a finding similar to studies that investigated the association between carotid IMT and current [63] and past [64] levels of leisure physical activity. The mechanisms behind this gender difference are not clear but may involve hormonal factors, differences in risk profile and arterial wall properties, but also different patterns and types of physical activity.

Current VO_2max was positively associated with femoral arterial compliance (i.e. buffering capacity) but not distensibility (i.e. elastic properties), a consequence of the much stronger association of VO_2max with femoral diameter than distension [12]. In athletes, as compared to sedentary peers, the diameter of the femoral (but not the carotid) artery is increased [65–67]. Our study showed that cardiopulmonary fitness was related to femoral arterial diameter even in adults without any special physical training, and that cardiopulmonary fitness at an early age may influence femoral arterial diameter much later. In contrast, and because of its relatively strong positive association with carotid arterial distension [12], current VO_2max was positively associated not only with compliance but also with distensibility of the carotid artery, suggesting that this artery underwent adaptations not only towards a higher buffering capacity but also towards a more elastic wall constitution. These associations were independent of, and thus unlikely to be mediated by, other cardiovascular risk factors. Adaptation to shear stress has been proposed to explain both the acute and the chronic changes of large artery properties to training-induced improvements of fitness [68–70]. During exercise blood flow increases (especially in arteries supplying the exercising musculature) leading to higher intraluminal shear forces, which stimulates the endothelium to release relaxing factors (e.g. nitric oxide) resulting in arterial vasodilation. In the long term, these repetitive increases in blood flow will result in arterial remodelling (i.e. larger vessel diameters), which occurs in order to restore basal shear stress. Other mechanisms may also play a role, such as a decrease in vascular smooth muscle tone as a consequence not only of an improved local and basal production of nitric oxide, but also of an exercise-induced reduction in sympathetic tone and/or renin-angiotensin system activity. A reduced resting heart rate, which is a known adaptation to endurance training, may also allow a more complete restoration of the arterial lumen diameter during the diastolic phase of the heart cycle, resulting in an increased buffering capacity.

Body Fatness, Body Fat Distribution and Carotid IMT and Arterial Stiffness

The positive and independent association between estimates of total and, for men only, central fatness during adolescence and carotid IMT at age 36 suggests that these risk factors can determine carotid wall thickening much later, which is in agreement with others [37]. At age 36, however, estimates of total and central fatness were not significantly associated with carotid IMT, which apparently contrasts with other studies [24, 26–30]. These studies have investigated other estimates of total and central fatness, such as the BMI and the waist circumference or the waist-to-hip ratio, which could explain the discrepancies. However, analyses in the present cohort at the age of 36 have shown that BMI and waist circumference were not significantly associated with carotid IMT in a linear fashion, but that carotid IMT was only significantly increased in the highest sex-specific tertiles of these estimates [36]. Nevertheless, accumulation of fat during adolescence seems to be particularly critical for adult arterial thickness. Considering that adolescence is a period characterized by fast growth and maturation, and where many lifestyles that may endure to adult age are acquired, the adolescent period may thus be a privileged window of opportunities for primary prevention [71, 72].

Total body fatness was inversely associated only with compliance of the femoral artery, which was due mainly to inverse associations with the distension of this artery (data not shown). However, this association decreased considerably after adjustments for fitness. Since fitness variables can also be intermediate variables (i.e. in the pathway between body fatness and arterial stiffness), the adjusted regression coefficients may thus underestimate the true associations between fatness and arterial stiffness. Central fatness, however, was independently and inversely associated not only with the compliance of the femoral artery but also with carotid distensibility and elastic modulus (positively) (i.e. the intrinsic elastic properties). This suggests that subcutaneous adipose cells may produce vasoactive mediators to which the carotid artery is particularly sensitive. Furthermore, the adaptations of the elastic carotid artery (but not the muscular femoral artery) as a consequence of increased subcutaneous truncal fat (but not overall adiposity) seem to have their roots already during adolescence. The elastic part of the arterial tree may thus be the first to be affected by the adverse effects of subcutaneous central fat. This study, as others [73], emphasizes that subcutaneous truncal fat may also have a deleterious effect on cardiovascular health, adding to the known deleterious effects of visceral fat. Since the associations between central fat and carotid IMT and large artery stiffness were independent of other risk factors, other mechanisms must thus explain these direct effects. The adipose tissue is an endocrine organ that produces many peptides, such as angiotensin, interleukin-6, tumor necrosis factor-α, plasminogen activator inhibitor-1, leptin and adiponectin [74], that in turn impact on vascular structure and function [75–77]. Regional differences in secretion of these peptides (e.g. higher in the trunk, either in the subcutaneous or visceral fat depot, than in the limbs) could thus explain the direct effects of subcutaneous truncal fat on arterial properties.

Fitness and Fatness Interactions in the Relationships with
Carotid IMT and Arterial Stiffness

We have shown that, overall, the associations between fitness and total and central fatness on the one hand and large artery properties on the other were independent of total and central fatness and fitness, respectively. In other words, despite being inversely related to each other, fitness and total and central fatness are not confounding the effects of total and central fatness and fitness on large artery properties, and are not intermediate variables (i.e. in the pathway) of these relationships.

The concept that proximal elastic arteries and peripheral muscular arteries respond differently to aging, drugs, and other factors is well established [77], and the present study suggests that the relative effects of fitness and adiposity, also, are not uniform along the arterial tree. In cross-sectional analyses, fitness seemed to be a stronger determinant of carotid stiffness whereas fatness seemed to be a stronger determinant of femoral stiffness. However, central fatness during adolescence was a stronger determinant of adult carotid IMT (in men) and stiffness (both men and women) than fitness. Taken together this suggests that some risk factors (i.e. central fatness) may be more critical than others (i.e. low fitness) at specific age periods (i.e. adolescence). Overall, our study does not allow the conclusion that fitness is a more potent risk factor than fatness or a central pattern of fat distribution (and vice versa), and that fitness attenuates the deleterious effects of fatness on central fatness or large artery structure and function. Therefore, our study, as that of the Lipid Research Clinic [46], does not support the findings from the

Aerobics Center Longitudinal Study [43–45], which includes exclusively men of the mid- to upper-socioeconomic strata. This limits the extrapolation of its results and may explain the discrepancies with other studies. Further investigation on this 'polemic' topic in other cohorts of both men and women, of different ethnicity and social backgrounds is thus warranted.

Conclusions

In conclusion, we show that both low levels of fitness and high levels of fatness can be deleterious for cardiovascular health, independently of each other and other risk factors. Moreover, our findings were not confined to highly fit or obese individuals but refer to a relatively young and asymptomatic free-living population of non-obese men and women. Thus, even moderate degrees of fitness and regional adiposity influence arterial structural and functional properties that are related to cardiovascular risk. Since some of these associations may have their roots in adolescence, and in view of the rising prevalence of obesity among children and adolescents, this study supports public health policies aiming at the improvement of physical activity levels and healthy diets early in life. Finally, it did not appear that being fit entirely attenuated the deleterious effects of being fat or that being slender entirely alleviated the effects of being unfit. Therefore, and in terms of implications for Public Health, the 'message' is that, to best preserve cardiovascular health, one must be fit *and* not (centrally) fat.

Acknowledgements

The first author of this paper is supported by a research grant from the Foundation for Science and Technology – Portuguese Ministry of Science and Technology (grant PRAXIS XXI/BD/19760/99).

References

1   Bots ML, Dijk JM, Oren A, Grobbee DE: Carotid intima-media thickness, arterial stiffness and risk of cardiovascular disease: Current evidence. J Hypertens 2002;20:2317–2325.
2   O'Rourke MF, Staessen JA, Vlachopoulos C, Duprez D, Plante GE: Clinical applications of arterial stiffness: Definitions and reference values. Am J Hypertens 2002;15:426–444.
3   Ross R: Atherosclerosis – An inflammatory disease. N Engl J Med 1999;340:115–126.
4   Laurent S, Katsahian S, Fassot C, Tropeano AI, Gautier I, Laloux B, Boutouyrie P: Aortic stiffness is an independent predictor of fatal stroke in essential hypertension. Stroke 2003;34:1203–1206.

5   Boutouyrie P, Tropeano AI, Asmar R, Gautier I, Benetos A, Lacolley P, Laurent S: Aortic stiffness
    is an independent predictor of primary coronary events in hypertensive patients: A longitudinal
    study. Hypertension 2002;39:10–15.
6   Liao D, Arnett DK, Tyroler HA, Riley WA, Chambless LE, Szklo M, Heiss G: Arterial stiffness
    and the development of hypertension. The ARIC study. Hypertension 1999;34:201–206.
7   Blacher J, Pannier B, Guerin AP, Marchais SJ, Safar ME, London GM: Carotid arterial stiffness
    as a predictor of cardiovascular and all-cause mortality in end-stage renal disease. Hypertension
    1998;32:570–574.
8   Bots ML, Grobbee DE: Intima media thickness as a surrogate marker for generalised atheroscle-
    rosis. Cardiovasc Drugs Ther 2002;16:341–351.
9   Blair SN, Kampert JB, Kohl HW III, Barlow CE, Macera CA, Paffenbarger RS Jr, Gibbons LW:
    Influences of cardiorespiratory fitness and other precursors on cardiovascular disease and all-
    cause mortality in men and women. JAMA 1996;276:205–210.
10 Blair SN, Kohl HW, Paffenbarger RS, Clark DG, Cooper KH, Gibbons LW: Physical fitness
    and all-cause mortality. A prospective study of healthy men and women. JAMA 1989;262:
    2395–2401.
11 Blair SN, Kohl HW III, Barlow CE, Paffenbarger RS, Gibbons LW, Macera CA: Changes in
    physical fitness and all-cause mortality: A prospective study of healthy and unhealthy men. JAMA
    1995;273:1093–1098.
12 Ferreira I, Twisk JWR, van Mechelen W, Kemper HCG, Stehouwer CD: Current and adolescent
    levels of cardiopulmonary fitness are related to large artery properties at age 36: The Amsterdam
    Growth and Health Longitudinal Study. Eur J Clin Invest 2002;32:723–731.
13 Lakka TA, Laukkanen JA, Rauramaa R, Salonen R, Lakka HM, Kaplan GA, Salonen JT:
    Cardiorespiratory fitness and the progression of carotid atherosclerosis in middle-aged men. Ann
    Intern Med 2001;134:12–20.
14 Rauramaa R, Rankinen T, Tuomainen P, Väisänen S, Mercuri M: Inverse relationship between
    cardiorespiratory fitness and carotid Atherosclerosis. Atherosclerosis 1995;112:213–221.
15 Vaitkevicius PV, Fleg JL, Engel JH, O'Connor FC, Wright JG, Lakatta LE, Yin FC, Lakatta EG:
    Effects of age and aerobic capacity on arterial stiffness in healthy adults. Circulation 1993;88:
    1456–1462.
16 Tanaka H, Desouza CA, Seals DR: Absence of age-related increase in central arterial stiffness in
    physically active women. Arterioscler Thromb Vasc Biol 1998;18:127–132.
17 Tanaka H, Dinenno FA, Monahan KD, Clevenger CM, DeSouza CA, Seals DR: Aging, habitual
    exercise, and dynamic arterial compliance. Circulation 2000;102:1270–1275.
18 Berenson GS, Srinivasan SR. Emergence of obesity and cardiovascular risk for coronary artery
    disease: The Bogalusa Heart Study. Prev Cardiol 2001;4:116–121.
19 Baumgartner RN, Heymsfield SB, Roche AF: Human body composition and the epidemiology of
    chronic disease. Obes Res 1995;3:73–95.
20 Grundy SM: Obesity, metabolic syndrome, and coronary atherosclerosis. Circulation 2002;105:
    2696–2698.
21 Poirier P, Eckel RH: Obesity and cardiovascular disease. Curr Atheroscler Rep 2002;4:448–453.
22 Björntorp P: Body fat distribution, insulin resistance, and metabolic diseases. Nutrition 1997;13:
    795–803.
23 Freedman DS, Williamson DF, Croft JB, Ballew C, Byers T: Relation of body fat distribution to
    ischemic heart disease. The National Health and Nutrition Examination Survey I (NHANES I):
    Epidemiologic follow-up study. Am J Epidemiol 1995;142:53–63.
24 Ciccone M, Maiorano A, De Pergola G, Minenna A, Giorgino R, Rizzon P: Microcirculatory
    damage of common carotid artery wall in obese and non obese subjects. Clin Hemorheol Microcirc
    1999;21:365–374.
25 Stevens J, Juhaeri, Cai J, Evans GW: Impact of body mass index on changes in common carotid
    artery wall thickness. Obes Res 2002;10:1000–1007.
26 De Michele M, Panico S, Iannuzzi A, Celentano E, Ciardullo AV, Galasso R, Sacchetti L, Zarrilli F,
    Bond MG, Rubba P: Association of obesity and central fat distribution with carotid artery wall thick-
    ening in middle-aged women. Stroke 2002;33:2923–2928.

27 Karason K, Wikstrand J, Sjostrom L, Wendelhag I: Weight loss and progression of early athero-sclerosis in the carotid artery: a four-year controlled study of obese subjects. Int J Obes Relat Metab Disord 1999;23:948–956.

28 Takami R, Takeda N, Hayashi M, Sasaki A, Kawachi S, Yoshino K, Takami K, Nakashima K, Akai A, Yamakita N, Yasuda K: Body fatness and fat distribution as predictors of metabolic abnormalities and early carotid atherosclerosis. Diab Care 2001;24:1248–1252.

29 Yamamoto M, Egusa G, Hara H, Yamakido M: Association of intraabdominal fat and carotid atherosclerosis in non-obese middle-aged men with normal glucose tolerance. Int J Obes Relat Metab Disord 1997;21:948–951.

30 Lakka TA, Lakka HM, Salonen R, Kaplan GA, Salonen JT: Abdominal obesity is associated with accelerated progression of carotid atherosclerosis in men. Atherosclerosis 2001;154:497–504.

31 Danias PG, Tritos NA, Stuber M, Botnar RM, Kissinger KV, Manning WJ: Comparison of aortic elasticity determined by cardiovascular magnetic resonance imaging in obese versus lean adults. Am J Cardiol 2003;91:195–199.

32 Oren S, Grossman E, Frohlich ED: Arterial and venous compliance in obese and nonobese subjects. Am J Cardiol 1996;77:665–667.

33 Resnick LM, Militianu D, Cunnings AJ, Pipe JG, Evelhoch JL, Soulen RL: Direct magnetic resonance determination of aortic distensibility in essential hypertension: Relation to age, abdominal visceral fat, and in situ intracellular free magnesium. Hypertension 1997;30:654–659.

34 Giltay EJ, Lambert J, Elbers JM, Gooren LJ, Asscheman H, Stehouwer CD: Arterial compliance and distensibility are modulated by body composition in both men and women but by insulin sensitivity only in women. Diabetologia 1999;42:214–221.

35 Mangoni AA, Giannattasio C, Brunani A, Failla M, Colombo M, Bolla G, Cavagnini F, Grassi G, Mancia G: Radial artery compliance in young, obese, normotensive subjects. Hypertension 1995; 26:984–988.

36 Ferreira I, Twisk JWR, van Mechelen W, Kempen HCG, Seidell JC, Stehovwer CDA: Current and adolescent body fatness and fat distribution: Relationships with carotid intima-media thickness and large artery stiffness at the age of 36 years. J Hypertens 2003; [in press].

37 McGill HC Jr, McMahan CA, Herderick EE, Zieske AW, Malcom GT, Tracy RE, Strong JP: Obesity accelerates the progression of coronary atherosclerosis in young men. Circulation 2002; 105:2712–2718.

38 Levent E, Goksen D, Ozyurek AR, Darcan S, Mahmut C, Coker M, Guven H, Parlar A: Stiffness of the abdominal aorta in obese children. J Pediatr Endocrinol Metab 2002;15:405–409.

39 Tounian P, Aggoun Y, Dubern B, Varille V, Guy-Grand B, Sidi D, Girardet JP, Bonnet D: Presence of increased stiffness of the common carotid artery and endothelial dysfunction in severely obese children: A prospective study. Lancet 2001;358:1400–1404.

40 Singhal A, Farooqi IS, Cole TJ, O'Rahilly S, Fewtrell M, Kattenhorn M, Lucas A, Deanfield J: Influence of leptin on arterial distensibility: A novel link between obesity and cardiovascular disease? Circulation 2002;106:1919–1924.

41 Malina RM, Beunen GP, Classens AL, Lefevre J, Vanden Eynde BV, Renson R, Vanreusel B, Simons J: Fatness and physical fitness of girls 7 to 17 years. Obes Res 1995;3:221–231.

42 Twisk JWR, Kemper HCG, van Mechelen W, Post GB, van Lenthe FJ: Body fatness: longitudinal relationship of body mass index and the sum of skinfolds with other risk factors for coronary heart disease. Int J Obes Relat Metab Disord 1998;22:915–922.

43 Church TS, Finley CE, Earnest CP, Kampert JB, Gibbons LW, Blair SN: Relative associations of fitness and fatness to fibrinogen, white blood cell count, uric acid and metabolic syndrome. Int J Obes Relat Metab Disord 2002;26:805–813.

44 Wei M, Kampert JB, Barlow CE, Nichaman MZ, Gibbons LW, Paffenbarger RS, Blair SN: Relationship between low cardiorespiratory fitness and mortality in normal-weight, overweight, and obese men. JAMA 1999;282:1547–1553.

45 Lee CD, Blair SN, Jackson AS: Cardiorespiratory fitness, body composition, and all-cause and cardiovascular disease mortality in men. Am J Clin Nutr 1999;69:373–380.

46 Stevens J, Cai J, Evenson KR, Thomas R: Fitness and fatness as predictors of mortality from all causes and from cardiovascular disease in men and women in the lipid research clinics study. Am J Epidemiol 2002;156:832–841.

47   van Lenthe FJ, Kemper HCG, van Mechelen W, Twisk JWR: Development and tracking of central patterns of subcutaneous fat in adolescence and adulthood: The Amsterdam Growth and Health Study. Int J Epidemiol 1996;25:1162–1171.

48   Kemper HCG, Twisk JWR, Koppes LLJ, van Mechelen W, Post GB: A 15-year physical activity pattern is positively related to aerobic fitness in young males and females (13–27 years). Eur J Appl Physiol 2001;84:395–402.

49   Welsman JR, Armstrong N, Nevill AM, Winter EM, Kirby BJ: Scaling peak VO_2 for differences in body size. Med Sci Sports Exerc 1996;28:259–265.

50   Weiner JS, Lourie JA (eds): Human Biology: A Guide to Field Methods. IBP Handbook No.9. Oxford, Blackwell, 1968.

51   Brands PJ, Hoeks APG, Willigers J, Willekes C, Reneman RS: An integrated system for the non-invasive assessment of vessel wall and hemodynamic properties of large arteries by means of ultrasound. Eur J Ultrasound 1999;9:257–266.

52   Reneman RS, Hoeks AP: Noninvasive vascular ultrasound: An asset in vascular medicine. Cardiovasc Res 2000;45:27–35.

53   Van Bortel LM, Duprez D, Starmans-Kool MJ, Safar ME, Giannattasio C, Cockcroft J, Kaiser DR, Thuillez C: Clinical applications of arterial stiffness, Task Force III: Recommendations for user procedures. Am J Hypertens 2002;15:445–452.

54   Van Bortel LM, Balkestein EJ, van der Heijden-Spek JJ, Vanmolkot FH, Staessen JA, Kragten JA, Vredeveld JW, Safar ME, Struijker Boudier HA, Hoeks AP: Non-invasive assessment of local arterial pulse pressure: Comparison of applanation tonometry and echo-tracking. J Hypertens 2001;19:1037–1044.

55   Bakker I, Twisk JWR, van Mechelen W, Mensink GB, Kemper HCG: Computerization of a dietary history interview in a running cohort; evaluation within the Amsterdam Growth and Health Longitudinal Study. Eur J Clin Nutr 2003;57:394–404.

56   Anderson JT, Jacobs DR Jr, Foster N, Hall Y, Moss D, Mojonnier L, Blackburn H: Scoring systems for evaluating dietary pattern effect on serum cholesterol. Prev Med 1979;8:525–537.

57   Tanaka H, Seals DR, Monahan KD, Clevenger CM, DeSouza CA, Dinenno FA: Regular aerobic exercise and the age-related increase in carotid artery intima-media thickness in healthy men. J Appl Physiol 2002;92:1458–1464.

58   Pauletto P, Palatini P, Da Ros S, Pagliara V, Santipolo N, Baccillieri S, Casiglia E, Mormino P, Pessina AC: Factors underlying the increase in carotid intima-media thickness in borderline hypertensives. Arterioscler Thromb Vasc Biol 1999;19:1231–1237.

59   Mayet J, Stanton AV, Chapman N, Foale RA, Hughes AD, Thom SA: Is carotid artery intima-media thickening a reliable marker of early atherosclerosis? J Cardiovasc Risk 2002;9:77–81.

60   Sader MA, Griffiths KA, McCredie RJ, Handelsman DJ, Celermajer DS: Androgenic anabolic steroids and arterial structure and function in male bodybuilders. J Am Coll Cardiol 2001;37:224–230.

61   Miyachi M, Donato AJ, Yamamoto K, Takahashi K, Gates PE, Moreau KL, Tanaka H: Greater age-related reductions in central arterial compliance in resistance-trained men. Hypertension 2003;41:130–135.

62   Schmidt-Trucksass A, Schmid A, Dorr B, Huonker M: The relationship of left ventricular to femoral artery structure in male athletes. Med Sci Sports Exerc 2003;35:214–219.

63   Stensland-Bugge E, Bønaa KH, Joakimsen O: Age and sex differences in the relationship between inherited and lifestyle risk factors and subclinical carotid atherosclerosis: The Tromso study. Atherosclerosis 2001;154:437–448.

64   Stensland-Bugge E, Bønaa KH, Joakimsen O, Njølstad I: Sex differences in the relationship of risk factors to subclinical carotid atherosclerosis measured 15 years later: The Tromso study. Stroke 2000;31:574–581.

65   Dinenno FA, Tanaka H, Monahan KD, Clevenger CM, Eskurza I, DeSouza CA, Seals DR: Regular endurance exercise induces expansive arterial remodelling in the trained limbs of healthy men. J Physiol (Lond) 2001;534:287–295.

66   Kool MJF, Struijker-Boudier HA, Wijnen JA, Hoeks APG, van Bortel LM: Effects of diurnal variability and exercise training on properties of large arteries. J Hypertens 1992;10: S49–S52.

67   Schmidt-Trucksass A, Schmid A, Brunner C, Scherer N, Zach G, Keul J, Huonker M: Arterial properties of the carotid and femoral artery in endurance-trained and paraplegic subjects. J Appl Physiol 2000;89:1956–1963.
68   Huonker M, Halle M, Keul J: Structural and functional adaptations of the cardiovascular system by training. Int J Sports Med 1996;17:S164–S172.
69   Shephard RJ, Balady GJ: Exercise as cardiovascular therapy. Circulation 1999;99:963–972.
70   Niebauer J, Cooke JP: Cardiovascular effects of exercise: Role of endothelial shear stress. J Am Coll Cardiol 1996;28:1652–1660.
71   Ebbeling CB, Pawlak DB, Ludwig DS: Childhood obesity: Public health crisis, common sense cure. Lancet 2002;360:473–482.
72   Williams CL, Hayman LL, Daniels SR, Robinson TN, Steinberger J, Paridon S, Bazzarre T: Cardiovascular health in childhood: A statement for health professionals from the Committee on Atherosclerosis, Hypertension, and Obesity in the Young (AHOY) of the Council on Cardiovascular Disease in the Young: American Heart Association. Circulation 2002;106:143–160.
73   Abate N, Garg A, Peshock RM, Stray-Gundersen J, Grundy SM: Relationships of generalized and regional adiposity to insulin sensitivity in men. J Clin Invest 1995;96:88–98.
74   Trayhurn P, Beattie JH: Physiological role of adipose tissue: White adipose tissue as an endocrine and secretory organ. Proc Nutr Soc 2001;60:329–339.
75   Ciccone M, Vettor R, Pannacciulli N, Minenna A, Bellacicco M, Rizzon P, Giorgino R, De Pergola G: Plasma leptin is independently associated with the intima-media thickness of the common carotid artery. Int J Obes Relat Metab Disord 2001;25:805–810.
76   Okamoto Y, Arita Y, Nishida M, Muraguchi M, Ouchi N, Takahashi M, Igura T, Inui Y, Kihara S, Nakamura T, Yamashita S, Miyagawa J, Funahashi T, Matsuzawa Y: An adipocyte-derived plasma protein, adiponectin, adheres to injured vascular walls. Horm Metab Res 2000;32:47–50.
77   Hak AE, Stehouwer CD, Bots ML, Polderman KH, Schalkwijk CG, Westendorp IC, Hofman A, Witteman JC: Associations of C-reactive protein with measures of obesity, insulin resistance, and subclinical atherosclerosis in healthy, middle-aged women. Arterioscler Thromb Vasc Biol 1999;19:1986–1991.
78   O'Rourke MF, Mancia G: Arterial stiffness. J Hypertens 1999;17:1–4.

Prof. Dr. Han C.G. Kemper
AGAHLS Research Group, EMGO-Institute
VU University Medical Center
Van der Boechorststraat 7, NL–1081 BT Amsterdam (The Netherlands)
Tel. +31 20 4448407; Fax +31 20 4446775, E-Mail hcg.kemper.emgo@med.vu.nl

Kemper HCG (ed): Amsterdam Growth and Health Longitudinal Study.
Med Sport Sci. Basel, Karger, 2004, vol 47, pp 101–122

....

Genetic and Environmental Factors in Relation to Adult Lumbar Bone Health

*Ingrid Bakker[a], Han C.G. Kemper[a], Jos W.R. Twisk[a],
Willem van Mechelen[a,b]*

[a] Institute for Research in Extramural Medicine (EMGO Institute), and
[b] Department of Social Medicine and Research Centre 'Body@Work' TNO VU,
     VU University Medical Center (Vumc), Amsterdam, The Netherlands

Abstract

Background/Aims: It was hypothesized that adult lumbar bone mineral density (LBMD) in males and females is related to genetic and environmental factors. In a longitudinal study the effects of genetic and environmental factors on LBMD over a 10-year period in adulthood (27–36 years of age) was studied. *Methods:* Vitamin D receptor (VDR) gene, estrogen receptor-α (ERα) gene, and the collagen type I alpha 1 (COLIA1) gene were the genetic factors studied. Physical activity, nutrition, and body composition were included as environmental factors to be studied. *Results:* A genetic relationship with adult LBMD was found for the *Pvu*II-*Xba*I polymorphism in the ERα gene. A positive longitudinal relationship between LBMD and the mechanical component of physical activity was demonstrated in males. From the 11 nutritional factors, LBMD was negatively associated only with fiber intake in males, and positively with alcohol consumption in females. Of the nine body composition components, fat-free mass (FFM) explained most of the variance in LBMD (4%) in both sexes. Gene-environment interactions were found for calcium intake with haplotypes of the VDR gene and for FFM with genotypes of the COLIA1 gene. *Conclusion:* Genetics (ERα gene) and environmental factors (physical activity, fiber, alcohol, and FFM) were related to LBMD in healthy Dutch adult males and females. The association of calcium intake and FFM with adult LBMD depends on the genotype.

Osteoporosis, a common worldwide health problem, is a multi-factorial disorder. Despite the considerable influence of heredity, bone health also depends on a whole range of environmental influences, which give the opportunity to alter these with positive benefits on osteoporosis or fracture risk. Environmental factors that contribute to the causes of osteoporosis later in life

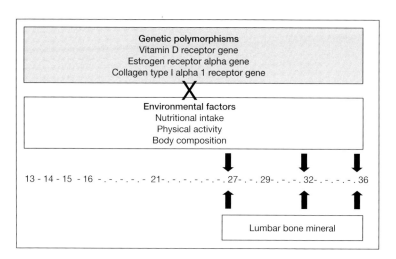

Fig. 1. Study design: the longitudinal relationship between genetics and environmental factors, and lumbar bone mineral density during adulthood (27–36 years), including the interaction between genetics and environmental factors in the longitudinal relationship.

include nutrition, hormones like estrogen, physical activity, body composition, alcohol consumption, and smoking habits [1]. None of these factors has a universal protective effect on developing osteoporosis.

Both genetics and environment contribute to the regulation of bone quality. They are known to influence the peak bone mass, which is reached in the late twenties, and probably the rate of loss of bone mineral at adult age and during elderly. Also of major interest are the possible gene-environment interactions. Knowledge on these interactions would give health care providers the possibility to adapt preventive and/or curative strategies against osteoporosis on the subjects' genetic predisposition. Up to date, it has not been thoroughly examined what the sole and combined influence of genetics and environmental factors is on bone mineral at adult age. To examine this, we analyzed the longitudinal relationship between lumbar bone mineral density (LBMD) during adulthood (27–36 years) and genetics, environmental factors (physical activity, nutrition, and body composition), and their interaction during this adult period (27–36 years), as shown in figure 1.

Background

Genetics

From twin and family studies, it has been indicated that genetic factors account for between 50 and 85% of the variance in bone mineral density, depending on the site of interest [2]. Of all sites, the lumbar spine bone mineral density (LBMD) has been suggested to have the highest heredity [3]. Genetic variation in several genes has been thought to be responsible for this genetic contribution. The vitamin D receptor (VDR) gene, the estrogen receptor-α (ERα) gene, and the collagen type I alpha 1 (COLIA1) gene are potential regulatory and structural candidate genes, associated with BMD [4].

Vitamin D Receptor (VDR) Gene

The biochemical mechanism of the VDR gene on bone density is uncertain. The VDR mediates vitamin D action by binding the active hormonal form of vitamin D, and subsequently increasing or decreasing the transcription of target genes [5]. The active hormonal form of vitamin D is a central regulator of bone and calcium homeostasis. The VDR is therefore a good candidate for determining BMD [6].

Estrogen Receptor-α (ERα) Gene

The estrogen endocrine system has an important role in the regulation of BMD and the occurrence of osteoporosis, i.e. exposure to lower estrogen levels is associated with a decreased BMD and subsequently with an increased risk for osteoporosis. Estrogen exerts its effect primarily via the ERα gene [7–9].

Collagen Type I Alpha 1 (COLIA1) Gene

Type 1 collagen is the major protein component of the bone matrix. A guanine-to-thymidine (G-to-T) substitution at the binding site for the transcription factor Sp1 in the COLIA1 is described and investigated by others [10–12]. The polymorphism with the T allele in the Sp1 binding site, causes a reduced binding affinity for the Sp1 protein [13], and alteration in the production and structure of collagen leads to 'osteoporosis imperfecta' and reduced BMD [14].

Environmental Factors

Physical Activity (PA). In most studies PA is described in terms of energy expenditure, because most methods of PA assessment are based on the intensity, frequency, and duration of the activities. However, this metabolic expression of PA might not be suitable for evaluating the effect of PA on bone.

From animal experiments, in which mechanical loads of various cycles were applied to different skeletal sites, it has been suggested that adaptive modeling and remodeling of bone is sensitive to changes in dynamic loading, and not to changes in static loading. Second, these experiments showed that the response of bone to a period of dynamic loading is quickly saturated. Third, the response is higher when the rate of change in the loading is higher, and when the distribution of the loading is unusual [15, 16]. These findings have led to the assumption that only a few, rather short repetitions of PA that cause high mechanical loads will have a positive effect on human bones [17].

Nutrition

Nutrition plays an important role by its direct involvement in the development and maintenance of bone mass and indirectly by maintaining normal postural reflexes and soft tissue mass [18]. Approximately 80–90% of bone mineral content is comprised of calcium and phosphorus. Other dietary components, such as protein, iron, vitamins D, A and C are required for normal bone metabolism, while other ingested components as fat, fiber, caffeine and alcohol may also impact bone health [19].

Regardless of what a person's baseline risk for osteoporosis might be for genetic reason, good nutrition helps to reduce the risk, and poor nutrition increases it. Adequate nutrition, including sufficient calcium, can have several effects on bone health. Firstly, adequate nutrition can maximize ones potential peak bone mass. Second, it can preserve the bone mass one has achieved during growth. Third, it can help the skeleton to recover from possible periods of disability, injury or illness during life [1].

Because some of the nutrients are suspected to have indirect effects on LBMD by influencing the effect, metabolism or excretion of calcium, it is also important to investigate interaction between calcium and other nutrients in the longitudinal relationship with LBMD.

Body Composition

Body composition components are also thought to be important determinants of bone mineral accrual and maintenance [20–22]. Special interest exists in total body weight (TBW), standing height, body mass index (BMI), waist circumference, hip circumference, waist/hip-ratio, sum of four skinfolds, fat mass (FM), and fat-free mass (FFM). Since total body weight, known to be related to bone mineral [23, 24], is composed of fat mass (FM) and fat-free mass (FFM), it is interesting to identify which of these two components mainly contributes to this relationship. FFM can be interpreted as a proxy for muscle mass.

Gene-Environment Interaction

The mechanism through which genetics might exert substantial influence on BMD remains elusive and is likely to be modified by the presence of various environmental factors like calcium intake, physical activity and FFM. For example, an interaction between calcium intake and VDR genotype in the relationship with BMD has been described [25–28]. It has been suggested that the VDR-calcium interaction depends on the level of dietary calcium intake, and that the association between VDR genotype and bone loss depends on the level of calcium intake [26]. The mechanism to explain the association between calcium and BMD only for those with a certain VDR genotype is that they might have a functional defect in their intestinal vitamin D receptor, resulting in reduced calcium absorption efficiency [26].

In a study among men, an association between COLIA1 polymorphism and BMD and muscle strength was found. The authors suggested that he _____ in BMD ___ __ ____ _____ ____ _____, by differences in muscle strength [29].

These and other findings suggest that increasing calcium intake, fat-free mass (as a proxy for muscle mass) and/or physical activity may be important in maximizing one's genetic potential for achieving and maintaining BMD.

Methods

During the 24 years of the AGAHLS (including approximately 600 males and females), nine repeated measurements of several environmental factors took place, starting at mean age 13 until the mean age of 36 years [30]. At the mean age of 27 years, lumbar bone measurements of the subjects were included in the design, and repeatedly measured at ages 32 and 36 years.

Genetics

DNA Extraction and Genotyping. In our study, haplotypes of three common polymorphisms in the VDR gene are investigated: *Bsm*I, *Apa*I, and *Taq*I. Also haplotypes of two polymorphisms in intron 1 of the ERα gene are investigated by us: *Pvu*II and *Xba*I. Finally, we investigated the polymorphism (*T* or *G* allele) at the binding site for the transcription factor Sp1 in the COLIA1 gene.

Genotyping was performed on DNA extracted from peripheral venous blood samples using standard techniques. Genotyping for the polymorphisms of the VDR gene, the ERα gene, and the COLIA1 gene were carried out by using restriction fragment length polymorphism-polymerase chain reaction (RFLP-PCR)-based methods as described elsewhere [31–33]. To confirm the accuracy of the genotyping, 150 randomly selected samples were genotyped for a second time with the same method. No discrepancies were found. All samples were genotyped blind. The genotypes are named according the absence (capital letter) or presence (small letter) of the restriction enyzme recognition sites that are created or abolished by the polymorphism.

Environmental Factors

Physical Activity. Total PA was measured by means of a structured detailed interview, based on the questionnaire developed by Verschuur for the AGAHLS [34]. For all measurements, a standard form containing cues was used during the interview to record the habitual PA pattern, except for the PA assessment at the mean age of 36. Then, an identical interviewer-administered computer-assisted version of the PA interview, developed for the

AGAHLS, was used. For all repeated measurements, the preceding 3 months were used as a reference period.

The intensity, frequency and duration of all PA (at school, during courses, at work, at home, during leisure time, organized and unorganized sports, climbing stairs, and transportation), with a non-stop duration of at least 5 minutes and exceeding the level of intensity of 4 times the resting metabolic rate (RMR), were taken into account [35]. The activities were classified into 3 categories: light (4–7 times RMR, e.g. cleaning windows, riding a horse, volleyball), medium heavy (7–10 times RMR, e.g. climbing stairs, moving furniture, aquarobics) and heavy (>10 times RMR, e.g. running, swimming, rowing), based on values reported in the literature [36–41]. For the analysis, a standard RMR value was assigned to all activities in each of these categories, i.e. 5.5, 8.5 and 11.5, respectively. A sum score of all activities in all three levels was calculated as total RMR*minutes per week, i.e. the weighted metabolic activity score per week (METPA). METPA was used as an estimate of the mean daily PA energy expenditure for the year of measurement [42].

PA was expressed also in terms of its biomechanical ground reaction forces (GRF), as described by Groothausen et al. [43]. Based on the GRF, all measured activities were classified into four categories, according to which one of the following scores was assigned: 0 (GRF <1 * body weight, e.g. cycling, swimming), 1 (GRF between 1 and 2 * body weight, e.g. rowing, aquarobics), 2 (GRF between 2 and 4 * body weight, e.g. cleaning windows, riding a horse) and 3 (GRF >4 * body weight, e.g. basketball, indoor soccer, volleyball). A sum score, MECHPA, was calculated as the sum of all GRF scores. This measure is irrespective of the duration, intensity and frequency of the activity.

Nutritional Intake

The habitual food intake was measured by a detailed cross-check dietary history face-to-face interview method, based on the method developed by Beal [44] and Marr [45], and adapted for the AGAHLS [46, 47]. This method provides information about the habitual dietary intake of the subjects, using the preceding 4 weeks as a reference period. The interview comprises the entire range of foods and drinks as listed in the Dutch Food and Nutrition Table [48]. Only items that were consumed at least twice a month were recorded. The cross-check consisted of an additional check on the reported frequency and amounts of the consumed foods and drinks. Amounts were reported in household measures or grams and models like glasses, bowels, and spoons were used to illustrate common portion sizes. Plastic examples of fruit and potatoes were used to facilitate the estimation of weights of those food items. From this interview, the mean daily intake of the nutritional factors (total energy, fat, protein, calcium, protein-to-calcium ratio, fiber, iron, vitamin A, vitamin C, alcohol and coffee) was calculated for each measurement by use of the 1996 database from the Dutch Food and Nutrition Table [48].

For all measurements, a standard form containing cues to record the habitual dietary intake was used during the interview, except at the mean age of 36 years. Then, an identical interviewer administered, computer-assisted version of the interview was used. The agreement between the data of both dietary interview methods was sufficient enough to be used in the longitudinal analyses [49].

Body Composition Components

In order to assess the body composition components, anthropometrical measurements were performed according the guidelines of the International Biological Program [50].

Total Body Weight (TBW). Participants dressed in underwear had body weights measured on a spring balance scale (van Vucht, Amsterdam, the Netherlands). Weights were recorded to the nearest 0.1 kg.

Standing Height. Height was measured without shoes, with a Harpenden digital read-out, wall-mounted or portable stadiometer (Holtain, UK; van Rietschoten & Houwens, Rotterdam, The Netherlands) and recorded to the nearest 0.1 cm.

Body Mass Index (BMI). This index was calculated by dividing total body weight (kg) to the squared standing height (m^2).

Circumferences of Waist and Hip. Circumferences of the waist and hip were measured with a flexible steel tape (Martin circumeter, Franken & Itallie, Amsterdam, the Netherlands) and recorded to the nearest 1 mm.

Waist/Hip Ratio. This ratio was calculated by dividing the waist circumference (mm) to the hip circumference (mm).

Sum of Four Skinfolds. Thickness of four skinfolds, i.e. biceps, triceps, sub-scapular, and supra-iliac skinfold, were measured at the left side of the body with a Harpenden skinfold caliper (Holtain, UK; van Rietschoten & Houwens, Rotterdam, the Netherlands) [51]. Skinfold thickness was measured at standardized anatomic locations and recorded to the nearest 0.1 mm.

Fat Mass (FM). From the equations, developed by Durnin and Womersley [52], fat mass was calculated from the sum of the four skinfolds, gender and age.

Fat-Free Mass (FFM). As an alternative measure of muscle mass, though also including bone mass, FFM was calculated as total body weight minus FM.

Other Environmental Determinants

Smoking habits and use of birth control pills were measured by questionnaire in order to be able to adjust for these environmental factors. The amount of smoked tobacco was expressed in grams of tobacco per week, as described by Bernaards et al. [53] and used as a continuous variable. Use of oral contraceptives (yes/no) was considered as the best possible proxy of increased estrogen levels in this study.

Outcome Variable

Lumbar Bone Mineral Density. Bone mass measurements were performed by means of dual-energy X-ray absorptiometry (DEXA) at the lumbar spine (L2–L4). The Norland XR 26 (Norland Corp., Fort Atkinson, Wisc., USA.) was used for the measurements at the mean ages of 27 and 32 years, and the Hologic QDR-2000 (S/N 2513; Hologic, Inc., Waltham, Mass., USA) was used for the measurements at the mean ages of 32 and 36. An estimation of LBMD was made of each lumbar vertebral body L2–L4, from which the average LBMD was calculated. The DEXA machine was calibrated daily before each session began. The correlation between the Norland and the Hologic is 0.988 for the lumbar spine [54]. To account for the change to another, highly correlated, DEXA machine during the course of the study, standardized values (z-scores) against the mean LBMD of all measured subjects were used for each measurement. For the bone measurements at the age of 32, the subjects measured on the same machine were grouped together as z-scores were calculated.

Data Analysis

All longitudinal linear relationships with LBMD were evaluated by means of multi-level analysis (MLwiN, Version 1.10.0007, Centre for Multilevel Modelling, Institute of

Education, London, UK) [55]. Multi-level analysis was performed because repeated measurements (at the mean ages of 27, 32 and 36) are clustered within individuals, and are therefore not independent.

In addition to the intercept, the outcome variable LBMD, and the predictor environmental variable, the crude model also included a time variable. The adjusted model was extended by inclusion of gender and the other non-predictor environmental variables (i.e. PA, CI, and/or TBW). Parameter estimates were considered to be significant at $p < 0.05$. Interaction terms were used in the adjusted model to investigate possible effect-modification by gender. When the p value of interaction between gender and PA was <0.10, stratified analyses were performed for males and females. For the analyses on nutritional intake and the body composition components, it was decided to stratify a priori for gender.

Genetics

For analysis on the longitudinal relationship between genetic predisposition and the adult lumbar bone between ages 27 and 36 years, subjects were grouped according to genotype. For the genetic association analysis, we used three statistical models to analyze differences between groups: (1) additive allele-dose effect; (2) dominant effect, and (3) recessive effect. More detailed information is described elsewhere [56]. In the crude analyses, correction was made for gender only. In the adjusted model, the correction was extended by FFM, MECHPA, calcium intake, alcohol consumption, use of birth control pills, and tobacco consumption. Hardy-Weinberg equilibrium (HWE) was calculated according to standard procedures using the χ^2 analysis.

Environmental Factors

For analyzing the univariate longitudinal linear relationships between each environmental variable and LBMD, the environmental variable was included in the model as a standardized continuous variable.

Because alcohol and coffee consumption were not normally distributed, for these variables only analyses on quartiles of consumption were performed. For these analyses the non-consumers were considered as the reference group and the consumers were divided into three equally sized groups.

Results

Genetics

Allele Frequencies. Allele frequencies for each polymorphism are shown in table 1. There is no evidence of deviation from Hardy-Weinberg equilibrium for any of the polymorphisms (VDR: $p = 0.94$, ERα: $p = 0.30$, COLIA1: $p = 0.09$).

Recessive, Dominant and Allele-Dose Effects. Gender was not found to modify the relationship between the haplotypes and LBMD. Therefore, no stratified analyses were performed, but analyses were adjusted for gender.

Analyses on *baT, BAt* and *bAT* haplotypes of the VDR gene showed no significant recessive, dominant or allele-dose effect. Among the haplotypes *px, PX* and *Px* of the ERα gene, *PX* showed a significant dominant (adjusted: $\beta = 0.210$,

Table 1. Allele frequency of polymorphisms of vitamin D receptor (VDR) gene, estrogen receptor alpha (ERα) gene and collagen I alpha 1 (COLIA1) gene

Polymorphism	n	Frequency, %
VDR haplotypes		
baT	347	52
BAt	245	37
bAT	74	11
ERα haplotypes		
px	341	50
PX	264	39
Px	79	11
COLIA1		
G	580	85
T	104	15

p = 0.04) and allele-dose effect (adjusted: β = 0.134, p = 0.04) on adult LBMD. Compared to non-*PX* carriers, *PX* heterozygotes had a higher LBMD (adjusted: β = 0.189, p = 0.08), and *PX* homozygotes had the highest LBMD (adjusted: β = 0.253, p = 0.06). No recessive, dominant and allele-dose effect on adult LBMD was found for polymorphisms in the COLIA 1 gene. More results can be found elsewhere [56].

Environmental Factors

The characteristics of the men and women at their mean ages of 27, 32 and 36 years are shown in table 2.

Physical Activity

For men, a positive linear longitudinal relationship was found between MECHPA and LBMD (β ± SD = 0.092 ± 0.040; p < 0.001). After correction for total body weight and calcium intake, this relationship remained the same (β$_{adj}$ ± SD = 0.090 ± 0.040; p < 0.001). No linear relationship between MECHPA and LBMD was found for women (β$_{adj}$ ± SD = 0.023 ± 0.034; p = 0.19). Also no linear relationship was found between METPA and LBMD with non-stratified analyses (β$_{adj}$ ± SD = 0.010 ± 0.029; p = 0.51). More detailed information is described elsewhere [57].

Nutritional Intake

Most of the linear relationships (crude and adjusted) were not significant (data not shown). However, within the analyses on quartiles, a significant

Table 2. Characteristics of the study population: mean ± SD of used longitudinal data (outcome and environmental factors) of adult men and women at the mean ages of 27, 32, and 36 years

	Men			Women		
	27 years (n = 84)	32 years (n = 197)	36 years (n = 170)	27 years (n = 97)	32 years (n = 207)	36 years (n = 182)
Outcome						
LBMD, g/cm^2						
Norland	1.170 ± 0.158	1.158 ± 0.180[a]	–	1.143 ± 0.138	1.125 ± 0.134[c]	–
Hologic	–	1.121 ± 0.146[b]	1.111 ± 0.160	–	1.093 ± 0.113[d]	1.065 ± 0.120
Environmental factors						
Physical activity						
MECHPA (score)	5.2 ± 2.7	5.8 ± 3.0	9.5 ± 3.6	4.8 ± 2.5	5.3 ± 2.6	9.2 ± 3.9
METPA (MET/week)	2,909 ± 2,262	3,257 ± 2,347	5,817 ± 3,082	3,209 ± 1,895	3,343 ± 2,081	6,971 ± 4,400
Nutrition						
Energy, MJ/day	12.0 ± 2.8	12.5 ± 3.2	12.4 ± 3.1	8.9 ± 2.0	9.3 ± 2.0	9.7 ± 2.1
Fat, g/day	121 ± 36	122 ± 41	111 ± 37	91 ± 28	91 ± 28	87 ± 23
Protein, g/day	105 ± 24	110 ± 28	110 ± 29	85 ± 18	88 ± 17	87 ± 16
Calcium, mg/day	1,363 ± 549	1,376 ± 626	1,431 ± 607	1,152 ± 414	1,189 ± 417	1,256 ± 411
Calcium-to-protein ratio, mg/g	12.7 ± 3.2	12.1 ± 3.0	12.8 ± 3.3	13.3 ± 3.1	13.4 ± 3.0	14.3 ± 3.1
Fiber, g/day	24.7 ± 6.5	29.8 ± 10.1	30.2 ± 9.9	20.0 ± 4.6	25.4 ± 6.6	26.3 ± 6.4
Iron, mg/day	13.1 ± 3.1	15.3 ± 3.7	15.6 ± 4.1	10.7 ± 2.1	12.6 ± 2.6	14.2 ± 15.2
Vitamin A, µg/day	865 ± 393	1,120 ± 511	991 ± 1,538	671 ± 275	804 ± 424	697 ± 608
Vitamin C, mg/day	137 ± 57	151 ± 64	125 ± 74	128 ± 48	147 ± 55	118 ± 120
Alcohol, g/day	11.7 ± 14.0	14.6 ± 16.1	18.4 ± 19.7	7.2 ± 9.9	7.2 ± 9.3	10.2 ± 13.1
Coffee, cups/day	4.1 ± 3.3	3.8 ± 3.2	5.1 ± 3.4	2.8 ± 2.1	2.7 ± 2.3	3.2 ± 2.3

Body composition						
Total body weight, kg	75.5 ± 8.4	81.1 ± 10.1	83.6 ± 10.7	63.2 ± 7.9	65.3 ± 8.6	68.0 ± 10.3
Standing height, cm	183.0 ± 6.6	183.7 ± 6.2	183.8 ± 6.5	170.2 ± 6.2	169.5 ± 6.5	170.1 ± 6.4
Body mass index, kg/m^2	22.5 ± 2.2	24.0 ± 2.6	24.7 ± 2.7	21.8 ± 2.5	22.7 ± 2.7	23.5 ± 3.3
Waist circumference, cm	78.4 ± 6.0	82.8 ± 7.5	85.1 ± 8.0	67.7 ± 5.6	70.3 ± 6.4	73.2 ± 8.4
Hip circumference, cm	86.9 ± 5.5	89.8 ± 6.5	89.2 ± 7.2	85.8 ± 7.5	89.0 ± 7.8	89.4 ± 8.6
Waist/hip-ratio	0.90 ± 0.06	0.92 ± 0.05	0.95 ± 0.05	0.79 ± 0.07	0.79 ± 0.04	0.82 ± 0.07
Sum of four skinfolds, mm	36.3 ± 13.5	42.0 ± 16.9	46.8 ± 15.5	45.8 ± 16.5	51.9 ± 18.4	55.7 ± 19.5
Fat mass, kg	11.0 ± 4.0	15.6 ± 4.9	17.2 ± 4.7	15.9 ± 4.6	18.5 ± 4.9	20.0 ± 5.7
Fat-free mass, kg	64.5 ± 6.1	65.4 ± 6.3	66.4 ± 6.9	47.3 ± 4.9	46.7 ± 4.8	48.0 ± 5.4
Other environmental factors						
Tobacco, g/week	37.2 ± 65.4	19.5 ± 49.2	19.9 ± 49.3	20.7 ± 50.2	14.8 ± 39.1	14.5 ± 38.3
Oral contraceptives, % yes	n.a.	n.a.	n.a.	62%	56%	41%

[a,b,c,d] n = 146, 51, 149 and 58, respectively.

n.a. = Not applicable.

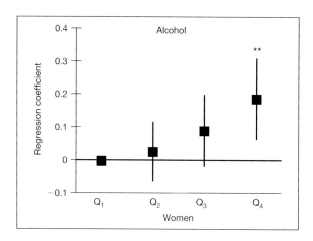

Fig. 2. Regression coefficients with the 95% CI for the longitudinal relationship for quartiles (Q_2–Q_4) of alcohol consumption and standardized (L2–L4) LBMD (g/cm^2) in women during adulthood (27–36 years), adjusted for total energy intake, MECHPA, FFM, tobacco consumption and use of oral contraceptives. With **p < 0.01.

difference with the reference group was found for alcohol consumption within women (fig. 2). Women within the highest quartile of alcohol consumption were found to have a significantly higher LBMD than women allocated to the reference group, i.e. non-alcohol consumers. Additional information can be found elsewhere [58].

Body Composition

The anthropometrical measures total body weight, BMI and FFM were significantly correlated to LBMD in the crude and adjusted univariate models for both sexes, and FM only for women. Significant adjusted linear regression coefficients of the anthropometrical measures are shown in figure 3. More detailed information can be found elsewhere [59].

Gene-Environment Interactions

Within the haplotypes of the VDR gene, effect modification by calcium intake was found. The effect of calcium intake on LBMD was however not significant for the VDR polymorphisms. In this, a non-significant positive effect was found for the intake of calcium on LBMD in *baT* heterozygotes ($\beta_{adj} = 0.094$ z-LBMD/g Ca; p = 0.06), while a non-significant negative effect of calcium intake on LBMD was found in the *baT* homozygotes ($\beta_{adj} = -0.062$ z-LBMD/g Ca; p = 0.31). The LBMD of *BAt* carriers were found also to be (non-significantly) positively associated with calcium intake ($\beta_{adj} = 0.087$

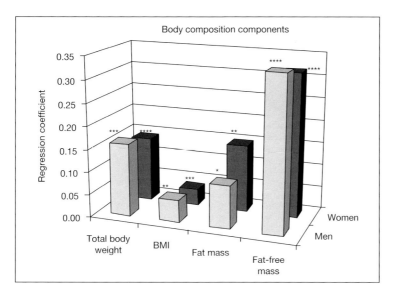

Fig. 3. Regression coefficients for the longitudinal relationship between the significant body composition components and standardized (L2–L4) LBMD (g/cm^2) during adulthood (27–36 years), adjusted for MECHPA and calcium intake. With *$p < 0.05$, **$p < 0.01$, ***$p < 0.001$, ****$p \leq 0.0001$.

z-LBMD/g Ca; $p = 0.06$). Interestingly, the polymorphism that is heterozygous for *baT* and carrier of *BAt* (*baT.BAt*), is the most common polymorphism in our study group (n = 136). In this group, a significant positive relationship between calcium intake and LBMD was found ($\beta_{adj} = 0.129$ z-LBMD/g Ca; $p = 0.02$).

No environmental effect modifiers could be detected for the relationship between ER haplotypes and LBMD.

Interestingly, FFM was found to modify the relationship between COLIA1 polymorphisms and LBMD ($p = 0.02$). The significant positive effect of FFM on LBMD ($p < 0.001$) in subjects carrying the *TT* genotype ($\beta_{adj} = 0.092$) was found to be higher than in *GT* ($\beta_{adj} = 0.036$) and *GG* ($\beta_{adj} = 0.029$) subjects. Figures 4a–c summarize the longitudinal relationship of the environmental factor (calcium intake and FFM) given a certain (group) of polymorphism(s), on the LBMD over the 10-year adult period.

Discussion

It was hypothesized that the prediction of LBMD at adult age not only depends on genetics but also on environmental factors, like physical activity, nutritional intake, and body composition.

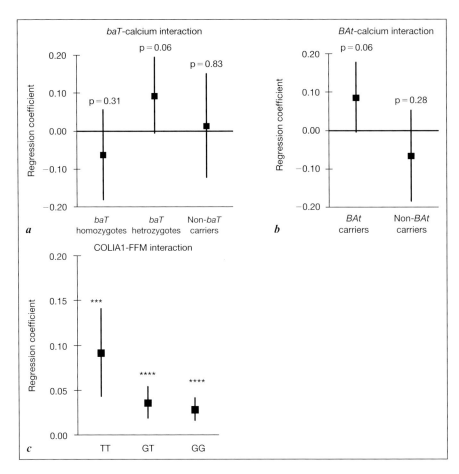

Fig. 4. *a* Regression coefficients for the longitudinal relationship between the calcium intake (g) and standardized (L2–L4) LBMD (g/cm²) in *baT* homozygotes, *baT* heterozygotes, and non-*baT* carriers of the VDR haplotypes during adulthood (27–36 years), adjusted for gender, FFM, MECHPA, total energy intake, alcohol consumption, tobacco consumption and use of birth control pills. *b* Regression coefficients for the longitudinal relationship between the calcium intake (g) and standardized (L2–L4) LBMD (g/cm²) in *BAt*-carriers and non-*BAt* carriers of the VDR haplotypes during adulthood (27–36 years), adjusted for gender, FFM, MECHPA, total energy intake, alcohol consumption, tobacco consumption and use of birth control pills. *c* Regression coefficients for the longitudinal relationship between the fat-free mass (kg) and standardized (L2–L4) LBMD (g/cm²) in *TT*, *GT*, and *GG* polymorphisms of the COLIA1 gene during adulthood (27–36 years), adjusted for gender, MECHPA, calcium intake, total energy intake, alcohol consumption, tobacco consumption and use of birth control pills. ***p < 0.001, ****p ≤ 0.0001.

Genetics

A pure genetic effect was only detected for the *PX*-polymorphism of the ERα gene. Men and women carrying this haplotype showed a positive relationship with LBMD at (young) adult age, with an increasing effect per number of *PX* alleles.

VDR Gene. Our analyses on the dominant and recessive effect of VDR haplotypes can be translated into those performed by others considering the *Bsm*I polymorphism only. No relationship between the VDR haplotypes and LBMD was detected in our study, while a meta-analysis including 16 papers, and performed in 1996, revealed that bone mass was lower in individuals with the *BB* genotype of the *Bsm*I polymorphism, compared to the *bb* genotype [60]. A difference in calcium intake between the different studies could explain this inconsistency [61]. In accordance with our results, but with *Bsm*I, *Taq*I and *Apa*I analyzed separately, Garnero et al. [62] showed that the VDR polymorphisms did not predict bone turnover or BMD in a sample of 189 healthy premenopausal French women (aged 31–57 years).

ERα Gene. Inconsistent associations of the ERα polymorphisms with BMD have been reported. In this, a mediating role for estrogen in the association between ERα polymorphisms and LBMD has been suggested [63]. In a population-based study of pre- and peri-menopausal women, *Pvu*II and *Xba*I ER genotypes were both separately associated with the levels of LBMD, i.e. a negative allele-dose effect for both *p* and *x* on LBMD, but not with the change in LBMD over a 3-year period [14].

Results from our study among (young) Dutch adult men and women, showing a positive relationship between the subjects carrying the *PX* haplotype and LBMD, are comparable to the studies only on *Pvu*II. The negative dominant *px* effect is equal to the *PP* effect. Therefore, in our study there was a positive trend ($\beta_{adj} = 0.179$, p = 0.09) between *PP* genotype and LBMD, while no relationship between *pp* and LBMD (i.e. recessive *px* effect) could be detected. For the allele-dose effect of *px*, and thereby also for *p* only, a negative trend was found with LBMD ($\beta_{adj} = -0.116$, p = 0.09). Our results are in agreement with the results found in the Rotterdam Study [32] and the Michigan Bone Health Study [14].

COLIA1. Like our study, the Michigan Bone Health Study, including 583 women aged 24–44 years, no relationship between COLIA1 polymorphisms and LBMD was identified [14]. However, Langdahl et al. [12] reported that subjects with the *TT* genotypes had significantly lower LBMD values than in subjects with the *GT* or *GG* genotypes. In the largest study to date, including 1,778 postmenopausal Dutch women, the effects of the COLIA1 polymorphisms on BMD were found to depend on age since menopause, suggesting a role in determining the rate of postmenopausal bone loss [10], and probably not during early adulthood.

Environmental Factors

Physical Activity. The magnitude of the linear regression coefficient indicates that a man with a 1 *sd* (approximately 3 units) higher score on MECHPA will have a higher LBMD of 0.09 *sd*. Because 1 *sd* in male LBMD is approximately 165 mg/cm^2, this means a 5 mg/cm^2 higher LBMD by one additional unit on the MECHPA score. This can be achieved, for example, by introducing jogging, skiing or golf in the PA pattern. However, when comparing the findings of the present study with the results reported in the literature, it can be argued whether such an increase in the MECHPA score is sufficient to achieve a relevant reduction in bone loss or an increase in LBMD. According to the relative risk for fractures described by Marshall et al. [64], an achievable increase of 0.1 *sd* in LBMD, resulting in a relative risk of 0.9 for fractures of the lumbar spine, might already be relevant.

No significant linear relationship was found between METPA and LBMD. Other studies investigating the relationship between the metabolic component of PA and LBMD, have reported significant positive linear relationships [25, 65], as well as no relationships [66].

Nutritional Intake

Almost none of the nutritional components showed a (significant) longitudinal relationship with LBMD over the period between the mean ages of 27 and 36 years. The nutritional component that showed a relationship with the development of (young) adult LBMD is alcohol in females. The alcohol consumption over the 10-year period of the subjects from the highest quartile is judged moderate (mean = 24 g/day; 5th to 95th percentile = 12–46 g/day). The relationship between calcium intake and LBMD development was found not to be masked by an interaction with another nutrient. Because this study was performed in healthy adults with overall a rather 'healthy' diet, this could at least partly explain why no relationship between nutritional intake and LBMD could be detected.

The requirement of dietary calcium is determined mainly by skeletal needs, and it exerts a threshold behavior. This means that adding more calcium above the threshold level (approximately 1,100 mg for adults), bone mineral is not likely to improve [67]. Overall, the mean daily intakes of both the males and females was far above this threshold level: 1,394 and 1,207 mg/day, respectively. This could explain why no relationship between calcium intake and LBMD was found.

Fiber is thought to influence the absorption of calcium inversely [68], but no significant interaction with calcium intake, nor a linear relationship with LBMD was found.

Moderate alcohol consumption appeared to be beneficial for bone. A suggested mechanism for the positive effect of moderate alcohol consumption in bone metabolism includes the induction of the production of androstenedione and its conversion into estrone, resulting in an increased estrogen concentration [69]. Another cause of increases in BMD with alcohol consumption that has been suggested is an increase in serum calcitonin concentration. In addition, serum parathyroid hormone and vitamin D metabolites are reported to be altered by alcohol consumption, which could cause a reduced bone resorption [70]. Moreover, alcohol has been shown to decrease the bone formation rate by decreasing the osteoblast number, osteoid formation, and osteoblast proliferation [71]. The combination of reduced bone resorption and decreased bone formation results in a reduced bone turnover or bone remodeling.

Why in the present study only a positive relationship between alcohol consumption and LBMD development was found for women and not for men, remains unclear.

Body Composition

The significant linear relationship between total body weight and the bone mineral measures can be explained partly by its gravitational effect on skeletal loading. This mechanism is not likely to be the principal mechanism for the relationship, since both its components FFM and FM would than expected to be independently related to bone mineral in both men and women [72], which was not true for FM in men. The relationship between total body weight and bone might therefore for a greater part be explained by only its major component, FFM, indicating a relationship concerning the force of muscle contractions on bone [23].

FM was only significantly related to LBMD in women. This fat-bone relationship can be explained by a number of mechanisms. The gravitational effect of soft tissue on skeletal loading might play a role, but also the association of FM with the secretion of bone active hormones from the pancreas and the secretion of bone active hormones like estrogens and leptin from the adipose tissue might be important [73].

The relationship between FFM and lumbar bone mineral suggests the importance of physical activity as a determinant of bone strength. And indeed, there was a relationship between physical activity expressed in metabolic equivalents and FFM. Thus, the relationship between FFM and bone mineral can at least partly be explained by mechanical stresses mediated through gravitational action and muscle contractions on bone [23].

Gene-environment Interactions

Effect modification by the environmental factors FFM and calcium was detected in the relationship between polymorphisms of respectively the COLIA1 and VDR genes and LBMD development. From the results of our study, it can be concluded that the influence of increasing calcium intake in adults is probably not always effective for LBMD. The effect of calcium on LBMD is likely to depend on the VDR polymorphism of the subject. Subjects not carrying the *baT.baT* polymorphism, but being heterozygous for the *baT* haplotype, and/or carrying the *BAt* haplotype are most likely to benefit from additional calcium. Further analysis on the subject carrying the *baT.BAt* polymorphism, which is the most common polymorphism in our study population (n = 136, 38%), indeed showed a positive relationship between calcium intake and LBMD ($\beta_{adj} = 0.129$, p = 0.02).

In our study, an interaction with FFM in the relationship between COLIA1 polymorphism and LBMD was observed. Results indicated that increasing FFM or muscle mass, was in all subjects related to an 'improvement' of adult LBMD, but the extend depends on the COLIA1 polymorphism of the subject. To our knowledge, no other study found an interaction between COLIA1 polymorphisms and FFM in the relationship with LBMD.

Conclusion

In summary, a pure genetic relationship with LBMD during the 3rd and 4th decade of life is found only for the *PX* polymorphism of the ERα gene, i.e. an allele-dose and a dominant effect. More interestingly are the gene-environment interactions found for the VDR gene in combination with calcium intake and for the COLIA1 gene in combination with FFM, which give health care providers the possibility to adjust preventive or curative treatment of osteoporosis to the genetic predisposition. Treatment with calcium is likely to have a positive effect in all non-*baT.baT* subjects, and in *BAt* carriers. The most common polymorphism in our group of Dutch subjects was the *baT.BAt*, which is also likely to benefit from extra calcium. Subjects carrying the *TT* genotype will benefit most from an increase in FFM.

We furthermore conclude that moderate alcohol intake appeared to have a positive relationship with LBMD development during adulthood for women in the highest quartile for alcohol consumption. Other nutritional components might also have had an impact on adult bone development, directly or via interaction with calcium, but the results were less pronounced, what might have been caused by the design of the study, including a 'healthy' population with a 'healthy' diet.

In addition, over the 10-year period, a significant positive linear relationship was found between PA, expressed in terms of biomechanical ground reaction forces (MECHPA), and LBMD during (young) adulthood (between 27 and 36 years of age) in males. For females no significant relationship between

MECHPA and LBMD was found for this 10-year period, although additional analyses on the first 6-year period showed a significant relationship. For the metabolic component of PA (METPA), no linear relationship with LBMD was.

From the nine investigated body composition components, total body weight, BMI, FM and FFM are positive associated with the 10-year development of bone mineral in adult men and women, of which FFM appeared to have the strongest relationship. Because FFM can be interpreted as a proxy for skeletal muscle mass, it is assumed that bone mineral is affected for a great part by mechanical stresses mediated through the force of muscle contractions on bone. Furthermore, because FFM represents the major component of total body weight, the relationship between FFM and bone mineral might also partly be explained by a gravitational effect.

References

1   Heaney RP: Bone mass, nutrition, and other lifestyle factors. Nutr Rev 1996;54:S3–S10.
2   Ralston SH: The genetics of osteoporosis. Q J Med 1997;90:247–251.
3   Cole DEC, Rubin LA: 1998 Osteoporosis and the interface between nutrition and genetics. Available at URL http://www.mcmaster.ca/inabis98/atkinson/cole0195/index.html
4   Gong G, Haynatzki G: Association between bone mineral density and candidate genes in different ethnic populations and its implications. Calcif Tissue Int 2003;72:113–123.
5   Ozisik G, Mergen H, Ozata M, Uyanik C, Caglayan S, Turan M, Boly E, Ilgin S, Oner R, Ozdemir IC, Oner C: Vitamin d-receptor gene polymorphisms and vertebral bone density in men with idiopathic hypogonadotrophic hypogonadism. Med Sci Monit 2001;7:233–237.
6   Morrison NA, Qi JC, Tokita A, Kelly PJ, Crofts L, Nguyen TV, Sambrook PN, Eisman JA: Prediction of bone density form vitamin D receptor alleles. Nature 1994;367:284–287.
7   Albagha OME, McGuigan FEA, Reid DM, Ralston SH: Estrogen receptor α gene polymorphisms and bone mineral density: Haplotype analysis in women from the United Kingdom. J Bone Miner Res 2001;16:128–134.
8   Kobayashi N, Fujino T, Shirogane T, Furuta I, Kobamatsu Y, Yaegashi M, Sakuragi N, Fujimoto S: Estrogen receptor alpha polymorphism as a genetic marker for bone loss, vertebral fractures and susceptibility to estrogen. Maturitas 2002;41:193–201.
9   Lau EMC, Young RP, Lam V, Li M, Woo J: Estrogen receptor gene polymorphism and bone mineral density in postmenopausal Chinese women. Bone 2001;29:96–98.
10 Uitterlinden AG, Burger H, Huang Q, Yue F, McGuigan FEA, Grant SFA, Hofman A, van Leeuwen JPTM, Pols HAP, Ralston SH: Relation of alleles at the collagen type I α1 gene to bone density and risk of osteoporotic fracture in postmenopausal women. N Engl J Med 1998;338:1016–1021.
11 Mann V, Hobson EE, Li B, Stewar T, Grant SFA, Robins SP, Aspden RM, Ralston SH: A COL1A1 Sp1 binding site polymorphism predisposes to osteoporotic fracture by affecting bone density and quality. J Clin Invest 2001;107:899–907.
12 Langdahl BL, Ralston SH, Grant SFA, Eriksen EF: An Sp1 binding site polymorphism in the COLIA1 gene predicts osteoporotic fractures in both men and women. J Bone Miner Res 1998;13:1384–1389.
13 Grant SFA, Reid DM, Blake G, Herd R, Fogelman I, Ralston SH: Reduced bone density and osteoporotic vertebral fracture associated with a polymorphic Sp1 binding site in the collagen type I α1 gene. Nat Genet 1996;14:203–205.
14 Willing M, Sowers M, Aron D, Clark MK, Burns T, Bunten C, Crutchfield, M, d'Agostino D, Jannausch M: Bone mineral density and its change in white women: Estrogen and vitamin D receptor genotypes and their interaction. J Bone Miner Res 1998;13:695–705.

15 Lanyon LE: Control of bone architecture by functional load bearing. J Bone Miner Res 1992; 7(suppl 2):S369–S375.

16 Lanyon LE: Using functional loading to influence bone mass and architecture: Objectives, mechanisms, and relationship with estrogen of the mechanically adaptive process in bone. Bone 1996;18(suppl):37S–43S.

17 Robling AG, Hinant FM, Burr DB, Turner CH: Shorter, more frequent mechanical loading sessions enhance bone mass. Med Sci Sports Exerc 2002;34:196–202.

18 Heaney RP: Calcium, dairy products and osteoporosis. J Am Coll Nutr 2000;19:83S–99S.

19 Reid DM: Nutrition and bone: Is there more to it than just calcium and vitamin D? Q J Med 2001; 94:53–56.

20 Edelstein SL, Barrett-Connor E: Relation between body size and bone mineral density in elderly men and women. Am J Epidemiol 1993;138:160–169.

21 Dawson-Hughes B, Shipp C, Sadowski L, Dallal G: Bone density of the radius, spine, and hip in relation to percent of ideal body weight in postmenopausal women. Calcif Tissue Int 1987;40: 310–314.

22 Glauber HS, Vollmer WM, Nevitt MC, Ensrud KE, Orwoll ES: Body weight versus body fat distribution, adiposity and frame size as predictors of bone density. J Clin Endocrinol Metab 1995;80:1118–1123.

23 Kroke A, Klipstein-Grobusch K, Bergmann MM, Weber K, Boeing H: Influence of body composition on quantitative ultrasound parameters of the os calcis in a population-based sample of pre- and postmenopausal women. Calcif Tissue Int 2000;66:5–10.

24 Harris SS, Dawson-Hughes B: Weight, body composition, and bone density in postmenopausal women. Calcif Tissue Int 1996;59:428–432.

25 Salamone LM, Glynn NW, Black DM, Ferrell RE, Palermo L, Epstein RS, Kuller LH, Cauley JA: Determinants of premenopausal bone mineral density: The interplay of genetic and lifestyle factors. J Bone Miner Res 1996;11:1557–1565.

26 Krall EA, Parry P, Lichter JB, Dawson-Hughes B: Vitamin D receptor alleles and rates of bone loss: Influences of years since menopause and calcium intake. J Bone Miner Res 1995;10: 978–984.

27 Ferrari SL, Rizzoli R, Slosman DO, Bonjour JP: Do dietary calcium and age explain the controversy surrounding the relationship between bone mineral density and vitamin D receptor gene polymorphisms? J Bone Miner Res 1998;13:363–370.

28 Kiel DP, Myers RH, Cupples LA, Kong ZF, Zhu XH, Ordovas J, Schaefer EJ, Felson DT, Rush D, Wilson PWF, Eisman JA, Holick MF: The *Bsm*I vitamin D receptor fragment length polymorphism (bb) influences the effect of calcium intake on bone mineral density. J Bone Miner Res 1997;12: 1049–1057.

29 Van Pottelbergh I, Goemaere S, Nuytinck L, De Paepe A, Kaufman JM: Association of the type I collagen alpha1 Sp1 polymorphism, bone density and upper limb muscle strength in community-dwelling elderly men. Osteoporos Int 2001;12:895–901.

30 Kemper HCG: Growth, health and fitness of teenagers: Longitudinal research in international perspective. Med Sport Sci. Basel, Karger, 1985, vol 20.

31 Uitterlinden AG, Pols HAP, Burger H, Huang Q, van Daele PLA, van Duijn CM, Hofman A, Birkenhäger JC, van Leeuwen JPTM: A large-scale population-based study of the association of vitamin D receptor gene polymorphisms with bone mineral density. J Bone Miner Res 1996;11: 1241–1248.

32 van Meurs JBJ, Schuit SCE, Weel AEAM, van der Klift M, Bergink AP, Arp PP, Colin EM, Fang Y, Hofman A, van Duijn CM, van Leeuwen JPTM, Pols HAP, Uitterlinden AG: Association of 5′ estrogen receptor alpha gene polymorphisms with bone mineral density, vertebral bone area and fracture risk. Submitted.

33 Uitterlinden AG, Burger H, Huang Q, Yue F, McGuigan FEA, Grant SFA, Hofman A, van Leeuwen JPTM, Pols HAP, Ralston SH: Relation of alleles at the collagen type I α1 gene to bone density and risk of osteoporotic fracture in postmenopausal women. N Engl J Med 1998;338: 1016–1021.

34 Verschuur R: Daily physical activity and health. Longitudinal changes during the teenage period; thesis, Universiteit van Amsterdam, SO 12, De Vrieseborch, Haarlem, 1987.

35 Kemper HCG, van Mechelen W: Methods and measurements used in the longitudinal study; in Kemper HCG (ed): The Amsterdam Growth Study: A Longitudinal Analysis of Health, Fitness and Lifestyle. HKP Sport Science Monograph Series, No 6. Champaign, Human Kinetics, 1995, pp 40–44.

36 Bink B, Bonjer FH, van der Sluys H: Assessment of the energy expenditure by indirect time and motion study; in Evang K, Lange Andersen K (eds): Physical Activity in Health and Disease. Oslo, Scandinavian University Books, 1966, pp 207–214.

37 Selinger V: Circulation responses to sport activities; in Evang K, Lange Andersen K (eds) Physical Activity in Health and Disease. Oslo, Scandinavian University Books, 1966, pp 198–206.

38 Durnin JVGA, Passmore R: Energy, Work and Leisure. London, Heinemann, 1967; Hollman W, Hettinger T: Arbeits- und trainingsgrundlagen. Stuttgart, Schattauer, 1976.

39 Reiff CG, Montoye HJ, Remington RD, Napier JA, Metzener HL, Epstein FH: Assessment of physical activity by questionnaire and interview; in Karvonen MJ, Barry AS (eds): Physical Activity and the Heart. Springfield, Thomas, 1976.

40 Lange Andersen K, Rutenfranz J, Masironi R, Seliger V: Habitual physical activity and health. WHO Reg Publ 1978, Eur Ser No 6.

41 Ainsworth BE, Haskell WL, Leon AS, Jacobs DR Jr, Montoye HJ, Sallis JF, Paffenbarger RS Jr: Compendium of physical activities: Classification of energy costs of human physical activities. Med Sci Sports Exerc 1993;25:71–80.

42 Montoye HJ, Kemper HCG, Saris WHM, Washburn RA: Measuring Physical Activity and Energy Expenditure, appendix P. Champaign, Human Kinetics, 1996, pp 182–183.

43 Groothausen J, Siemer H, Kemper HCG, Twisk JWR, Welten DC: Influence of peak strain on lumbar bone mineral density: An analysis of 15-year physical activity in young males and females. Pediatr Exerc Sci 1997;9:159–173.

44 Beal VA: The nutritional history in longitudinal research. J Am Diet Assoc 1967;51:426–432.

45 Marr JW: Individual dietary surveys: Purpose and methods. World Rev Nutr Diet. Basel, Karger, 1971, vol 13, pp 105–164.

46 Kemper HCG, van Mechelen W: Methods and measurements used in the longitudinal study; in Kemper HCG (ed): The Amsterdam Growth Study: A Longitudinal Analysis of Health, Fitness and Lifestyle. HKP Sport Science Monograph Series. Champaign, Human Kinetics, 1995, vol 6, pp 40–44.

47 Post GB: Nutrition in adolescence: A longitudinal study in dietary pattern from teenager to adult; thesis, Agricultural University Wageningen, SO 16, Haarlem, The Netherlands: De Vrieseborch, 1989.

48 van der Heijden LJM, Hulshof KFAM, Langius JAE, van Oosten HM, Pruissen-Boskaljon JC, van Stratum P: NEVO tabel, Nederlands Voedingsstoffenbestand 1996 (in Dutch) (Dutch Food Composition Table 1996). Den Haag, Voorlichtingsbureau voor de voeding, 1996.

49 Bakker I, Twisk JWR, van Mechelen W, Mensink GBM, Kemper HCG: Computerization of a dietary history interview in a running cohort: Evaluation within the Amsterdam Growth and Health Longitudinal Study. Eur J Clin Nutr 2003;57:394–404.

50 Weiner JS, Lourie JA: Human Biology: A Guide to Field Methods. Oxford, Blackwell, 1968.

51 Durnin JVGA, Rahaman MM: The assessment of the amount of fat in the human body from measurements of skinfold thickness. Br J Nutr 1967;21:681–689.

52 Durnin JVGA, Womersley J: Body fat assessed from total body density and its estimation from skinfold thickness: Measurements on 481 men and women aged form 16 to 72 years. Br J Nutr 1974;32:77–97.

53 Bernaards CM, Twisk JWR, Snel J, van Mechelen W, Kemper HCG: Is calculating pack-years retrospectively a valid method to estimate life-time tobacco smoking? A comparison between prospectively calculated pack-years and retrospectively calculated pack-years. Addiction 2001; 96:1653–1662.

54 Genant HK, Grampp S, Glüer CC, Faulkner KG, Jergas M, Engelke K, Hagiwara S, van Kuijk C: Universal Standardization for dual X-ray absorptiometry: Patient and phantom cross-calibration results. J Bone Miner Res 1994;9:1503–1514.

55 Goldstein H: Multilevel Statistical Models. New York, Wiley, 1995.

56   Bakker I, Uitterlinden AG, Twisk JWR, van Mechelen W, Pols HAP, Kemper HCG: Genetic determinants and gene-environment interactions in the 10-year longitudinal development of lumbar bone mineral in (young) adult men and women. Submitted.

57   Bakker I, Twisk JWR, van Mechelen W, Roos JC, Kemper HCG: 10-year longitudinal relationship between physical activity and lumbar bone mass in (young) adults. J Bone Miner Res 2003;18: 325–323.

58   Bakker I, Twisk JWR, van Mechelen W, Kemper HCG: Ten-year longitudinal relationship between nutrition and lumbar bone mineral density in (young) adult men and women. Submitted.

59   Bakker I, Twisk JWR, van Mechelen W, Kemper HCG: Fat-free body mass: The most important body composition determinant of 10-year longitudinal development of lumbar bone in (young) adult men and women. J Clin Endocrinol Metab 2003;88:in press.

60   Cooper GS, Umbach DM: Are vitamin D receptor polymorphisms associated with bone mineral density? A meta-analysis. J Bone Miner Res 1996;11:1841–1849.

61   Laaksonen M, Kärkkäinen M, Outila T, Vanninen T, Ray C, Lamberg-Allardt C: Vitamin D receptor gene *Bsm*I-polymorphism in Finnish premenopausal and postmenopausal women: Its association with bone mineral density, markers of bone turnover, and intestinal calcium absorption, with adjustment for lifestyle factors. J Bone Miner Metab 2002;20:383–390.

62   Garnero P, Borel O, Sornay-Rendu E, Delmas PD: Vitamin D receptor gene polymorphisms do not predict bone turnover and bone mass in healthy premenopausal women. J Bone Miner Res 1996; 10:1283–1288.

63   Turner RT, Riggs BL, Spelsberg TC: Skeletal effects of estrogen. Endocr Rev 1994;15:275–300.

64   Marshall D, Johnell O, Wedel H: Meta-analysis of how well measures of bone density predict occurrence of osteoporotic fractures. BMJ 1996;312:1254–1259.

65   Recker RR, Davie KM, Hinders SM, Heaney RP, Stegman MR, Kimmel DB: Bone gain in young adult women. JAMA 1992;268:2403–2408.

66   Kröger H, Tuppurainen M, Honkanen R, Alhava E, Saarikoski S: Bone mineral density and risk factors for osteoporosis: A population-based study of 1600 perimenopausal women. Calcif Tissue Int 1994;55:1–7.

67   Illich JZ, Kerstetter JE: Nutrition in bone health revisited: A story beyond calcium. J Am Coll Nutr 2000;19:715–737.

68   Weaver CM, Heaney RP, Martin BR, Fitzsimmons ML: Human calcium absorption from whole-wheat products. J Nutr 1991;121:1769–1775.

69   Holbrook TL, Barrett-Conner E: A prospective study of alcohol consumption and bone mineral density. BMJ 1993;306:1506–1509.

70   Rico H: Alcohol and bone disease. Alcohol 1990;25:345–352.

71   Klein RF, Fausti KA, Carlos AS: Ethanol inhibits hyman osteoblastic cell proliferation. Alcohol Clin Exp Res 1996;20:572–578.

72   Reid IR, Plank LC, Evans MC: Fat mass is an important determinant of whole body bone density in premenopausal women but not in men. J Clin Endocrinol Metab 1992;75:779–782.

73   Reid IR: Relationships among body mass, its components, and bone. Bone 2002;31:547–555.

Prof. Dr. Han C.G. Kemper
AGAHLS Research Group, Institute for Research in Extramural Medicine
VU University Medical Center
Van der Boechorststraat 7, NL–1081 BT Amsterdam (The Netherlands)
Tel. +31 20 4448407, Fax +31 20 4446775, E-Mail hcg.kemper.emgo@med.vu.nl

Kemper HCG (ed): Amsterdam Growth and Health Longitudinal Study.
Med Sport Sci. Basel, Karger, 2004, vol 47, pp 123–131

....

Smoking, Alcohol and Coffee Consumption and Cardiovascular Risk Indicators

Jan Snel[b], *Lando L.J. Koppes*[a], *Han C.G. Kemper*[a]

[a] EMGO Institute, VU University Medical Center, Amsterdam, and
[b] Department of Psychology, University of Amsterdam, Amsterdam, The Netherlands

Abstract

Background/Aims: The relationship between smoking, alcohol consumption and coffee and indicators of cardiovascular risk was assessed with the methods as described in the chapter by Koppes et al. [pp 44–63]. Coffee consumption was measured with a questionnaire asking for amount of coffee consumed over the day. CVD risk indicators were: serum total cholesterol (TC), high-density lipoprotein cholesterol (HDL-C), triglycerides (TG), systolic and diastolic blood pressure (SBP and DBP), the sum of 4 skinfolds (S4S), the waist-hip circumference ratio (WHR), and the maximal oxygen uptake/kg BW (VO$_2$max). ***Results:*** Smoking was associated with an increased cardiovascular risk (higher TC, lower HDL-C and lower VO$_2$max levels). Slightly more favorable profiles were found for alcohol use (higher HDL-C, higher dose-dependent VO$_2$max) and coffee drinking (slightly higher HDL-C and lower SBP). ***Conclusion:*** No smoking, moderate alcohol and coffee intake are weakly related with healthier levels of CVD risk indicators. In order to draw firmer conclusions, other factors should be taken into account such as motives for use of recreational substances, and the attitude and the emotions related to their use.

There is increasing evidence to suggest that the lifestyle components smoking [1–3] and alcohol consumption [4–6] have important relationships with cardiovascular disease. The American Council on Science and Health (ACSH) [7] refers to evidence showing that cigarette smoking in a dose-dependent way increases the risk of CHD for both men and women. In the Nurses' Health Study it was found that those who smoked daily at least 25 cigarettes had a 5.5 times higher risk of fatal CHD than non-smokers, while for those who smoked 1–4 or 5–14 cigarettes the risk was 2–3 higher. As for the consumption of alcohol the

ACSH admits that although moderate drinking may help the heart, more than 5.6 drinks of 10 gram alcohol per day (4 USA standard units) interferes with its mechanical functioning and over a period of years is responsible for 20–50 percent of cases of cardiomyopathy. Such heavy use when chronic or acute overconsumption may disturb the rhythm of the heart. Also, binge drinking, the episodic heave drinking, is associated with ischaemic stroke in men.

The association between coffee consumption and cardiovascular disease has been debated over a long period [8, 9]. In an extensive review Nawrot et al. [10] concluded that for the healthy adult population, moderate daily caffeine intake up to 400 mg day (3–5 cups of coffee) is not associated with adverse cardiovascular effects. Also clinical studies have shown that high acute doses up to 450 mg do not increase the frequency or severity of cardiac arrhythmias in healthy persons, ischemic heart patients or those with serious ventricular ectopia. As for heart rate the small decrease that is generally noted is probably clinically not relevant. Other CHD-related parameters such as cholesterol may show a small increase in the case that no paper filters are used. The clinical significance of the modest pressor effect of caffeine is still under discussion. The almost 60 studies that have been completed on blood pressure show in healthy users and hypertensives that with an acute dose of more than 250 mg (about 3 cups of coffee) SBP increases with 5–15 mm Hg and DBP with 5–10 mm Hg, but tolerance to this pressor effect occurs within 1–3 days. This latter aspect may be important as Lane et al. [11] showed. They found in 47 healthy, nonsmoking habitual coffee drinkers that during normal activities at work and at home in the evening a fixed dose of 500 mg (about 4–6 cups of coffee) decreased average BP with about 4 mm Hg and heart rate with 2 bpm. Interestingly, epinephrine levels increased on average 32%. A review of epidemiological evidence, however, made clear that there is no relationship between coffee use and BP [10].

The causal pathways through which tobacco, an alcoholic drink and coffee have their effects on cardiovascular health remain obscure. This is not surprising since next to the substances themselves, these consumer products not only contain hundreds of solid and volatile substances, but also non-nicotinic, non-alcoholic and non-caffeinic factors have their influence. Support for the idea that caffeine in coffee is not responsible for cardiovascular effects comes from epidemiological studies showing an increased risk of coronary events with consumption of decaffeinated coffee [12]. Also the experimental study by Corti et al. [13] with a within-subjects design in 6 habitual and 9 nonhabitual coffee drinkers indicated that a caffeinated or decaffeinated triple espresso or an i.v. dose of 250 mg induced comparable increases of sympathetic nerve activity and blood pressure (SBP: 12 mm Hg; DBP: 6 mm Hg).

An other critical comment on the literature is that hardly any notice has been taken of the amount of consumption not to mention the change of consumption. For these reasons, our goal was to investigate the relationships between the lifestyle behaviors smoking, alcohol and coffee consumption, and several risk factors for CVD. The assumption was tested whether no smoking and moderate alcohol and coffee consumption were related to healthier levels of the assessed CVD risk factors.

Methods

Variables Studied

In this chapter, we considered components of lifestyle as determinants of CVD risk indicators. The lifestyle behaviors are smoking, alcohol and coffee consumption. The AGAHLS assessment methods of alcohol and tobacco consumption are described in the chapter by Koppes et al. [pp 44–63]. Coffee consumption was assessed using a questionnaire asking for the number of cups of coffee consumed within eight periods of the day: Before, with, and after breakfast, with, and after lunch, before and with dinner, in the evening, and in the night. The CVD risk indicators are the serum concentration of total cholesterol (TC), high-density lipoprotein cholesterol (HDL-C), and triglycerides (TG), Systolic and Diastolic blood pressure (SBP and DBP), the sum of 4 skinfolds (S4S), the ratio of the circumference of the waist and hip (WHR), and the maximal oxygen uptake per kg bodyweight (VO$_2$max).

Analyses

Linear regression analyses were used in three ways to study the relationships between tobacco, alcohol and coffee consumption, and the CVD risk indicators.

First, the lifestyle variables at the age of 32 years were used as dichotomous determinants. With these analyses, the differences between consumers and non-consumers of tobacco, alcohol, and coffee with respect to the CVD risk indicators were elucidated.

Second, in consumers at age of 32 years cross-sectional relationships between the amount of tobacco, alcohol and coffee consumption, and CVD risk indicators were investigated.

Third, the scores of all variables of interest obtained at age 32 years were subtracted from those obtained at the age of 36 years. The resulting change scores from all participants were used to investigate the longitudinal relationships between 4-year changes in the amount of tobacco, alcohol and coffee consumption and the concomitant changes on the CVD risk indicators. The 7 participants who used CVD-related medication in the 12 months prior to one or both assessments were left out of all analyses. Interactions between the lifestyle variables and gender were analyzed, and if significant, stratified analyses were performed. If the interaction term was not significant, analyses were controlled for gender. Analyses for smoking, alcohol and tobacco consumption were additionally corrected for one another. In addition, potential confounding by (changes in) physical activity (METs/week) or dietary intake (kJ/kg body weight) was controlled for.

Results

Descriptive data of the tobacco, alcohol, TC, HDL, SBP, DBP, S4S, and VO$_2$max are shown in the chapter by Koppes et al. [pp 44–63]. At age 32 years,

Table 1. Regression coefficients (b) and 95% confidence intervals (CI) regarding the score on eight CVD risk factors, and (1) being a smoker of tobacco or not; (2) the amount of tobacco consumed by smokers, and (3) a change in the amount of tobacco consumption

	Age 32 years (yes vs. no) n = 322 (149 and 173)		Age 32 years (g/day) n = 57 (31 and 26)		Change 32 to 36 years (g/day) n = 310 (141 and 169)	
	b	CI	b	CI	b	CI
TC, mmol/l	M 0.43	0.08–0.78	0.01	−0.01–0.04	M 0.02	0.00–0.05
	W −0.07	−0.39–0.26			W −0.01	−0.03–0.02
HDL-C, mmol/l	−0.05	−0.14–0.04	−0.02	−0.03 to −0.01	−0.00	−0.01–0.00
TG, mmol/l	M 0.62	0.29–0.95	0.03	−0.00–0.07	0.01	−0.01–0.02
	W 0.17	0.02–0.33				
SBP, mm Hg	−1.72	−4.75–1.30	M 0.44	0.04–0.85	−0.23	−0.51–0.04
			W −0.78	−1.34 to −0.23		
DBP, mm Hg	−1.77	−4.06–0.52	0.09	−0.17–0.35	−0.19	−0.42–0.03
S4S, cm	0.13	−0.33–0.57	0.10	0.03–0.16	M 0.03	−0.00–0.06
					W −0.03	−0.07–0.01
WHR, %	1.29	0.14–2.45	0.07	−0.08–0.22	−0.15	−0.32–0.02
VO₂max, ml/kg/min	M −4.00	−6.53–1.44	−0.25	−0.47 to −0.03	−0.04	−0.18–0.11
	W −0.48	−2.72–1.76				

A consistent positive relationship was found between alcohol consumption and HDL-C (table 2). Drinkers had higher levels than non-drinkers. The more alcohol consumed, the higher the HDL-C, and a change in the amount of alcohol consumed was positively related with a change in HDL-C. Drinkers of alcohol further had smaller skinfold thicknesses, and a 2.9 ml/kg/min higher VO₂max. Women who consumed more alcohol had a lower DBP than women who consumed less alcohol. Finally, an increase in the amount of alcohol consumed was related with a borderline significant decrease of the WHR, and in men, with a highly significant 1.5 ml/kg/min increase in VO₂max.

77% of the men and women were consumers of coffee. These drinkers consumed an average of 4.8 and 3.6 cups per day, respectively. Over the following 4 years, this percentage of coffee drinkers showed a 15 increase in men, and 9 in women. The amount of coffee per drinker increased as well, with 0.8 cups per day in men, and with 0.2 cups per day in women. The mean serum concentration of TG was higher in men than in women (at the age of 32 years, 1.27 and 0.92 mmol/l, respectively). Over the following 4 years, TG also increased more in men than in women (0.26 and 0.03 mmol/l, respectively). At the age of 32 years, the WHR was higher in men than in women (92 vs. 79%). Over the following 4 years, a WHR increase of 3% was seen in both sexes.

Table 2. Regression coefficients (b) and 95% confidence intervals (CI) regarding the score on eight CVD risk factors, and (1) being a drinker of alcohol or not; (2) the amount of alcohol consumed by drinkers, and (3) a change in the amount of alcohol consumption

	Age 32 years (yes vs. no) n = 322 (149 and 173)		Age 32 years (10 g Unit per day) n = 253 (129 and 125)		Change 32–36 years (10 g Unit per day) n = 310 (141 and 169)	
	b	CI	b	CI	b	CI
TC, mmol/l	0.10	−0.14–0.35	0.05	−0.05–0.14	0.02	−0.04–0.08
HDL-C, mmol/l	0.09	0.00–0.18	0.04	0.01–0.08	0.05	0.03–0.07
TG, mmol/l	0.00	−0.18–0.19	−0.03	−0.10–0.05	−0.03	−0.10–0.04
SBP, mm Hg	−1.46	−4.58–1.67	0.01	−1.25–1.26	−0.28	−1.35–0.79
DBP, mm Hg	0.15	−2.22–2.51	M 0.25	−0.83–1.32	0.17	−0.71–1.05
			W −2.23	−4.35 to −0.10		
S4S, cm	−0.54	−1.01 to −0.08	−0.01	−0.18–0.16	0.01	−0.09–0.11
WHR, %	0.29	−0.90–1.48	0.24	−0.24–0.71	−0.65	−1.30–0.01
VO$_2$max, ml/kg/min	M −0.84	−4.26–2.58	−0.13	−0.82–0.55	M 1.53	0.64–2.43
	W 2.94	1.00–4.88			W −0.05	−0.49–0.40

As for the consumption of coffee and its relationship to CVD risk factors only two relationships were statistically significant (table 3). First, consumers who drank more coffee at age 32 years had lower SBP values than those who drank less coffee. Per additional cup per day SBP values were 0.6 mm Hg lower. Second, a change in the amount of coffee consumption was found positively related with a change in HDL-C (p = 0.02). Post-hoc analyses revealed that this longitudinal relationship was due to the HDL-C change related with the four-year change in the amount of coffee consumption in drinkers, and not to the change in HDL-C levels in participants who had started or stopped drinking coffee between the ages of 32 and 36 years.

Table 3. Regression coefficients (b) and 95% confidence intervals (CI) regarding the score on eight CVD risk factors, and (1) being a coffee drinker or not; (2) the amount of coffee consumed by drinkers, and (3) a change in the amount of coffee consumption

	Age 32 years (yes vs. no) n = 322 (149 and 173)		Age 32 years (cups per day) (n = 240)		Change 32–36 years (cups per day) n = 310 (141 and 169)	
	b	CI	b	CI	b	CI
TC, mmol/l	−0.05	−0.27–0.17	0.03	−0.02–0.08	−0.00	−0.03–0.02
HDL-C, mmol/l	−0.08	−0.16–0.01	0.01	−0.00–0.03	0.01	0.00–0.02
TG, mmol/l	0.09	−0.09–0.25	−0.02	−0.06–0.02	−0.01	−0.04–0.02
SBP, mm Hg	1.68	−1.15–4.51	−0.63	−1.23 to −0.03	−0.22	−0.70–0.26
DBP, mm Hg	1.21	−0.94–3.35	−0.21	−0.67–0.25	−0.14	−0.53–0.25
S4S, cm	−0.18	−0.60–0.25	−0.01	−0.10–0.08	−0.02	−0.07–0.02
WHR, %	0.38	−0.70–1.46	−0.08	−0.31–0.15	0.21	−0.08–0.51
VO$_2$max, ml/kg/min	−0.03	−1.65–1.59	−0.12	−0.46–0.22	−0.02	−0.29–0.23

After controlling for gender, alcohol and coffee consumption, physical activity and dietary energy intake (table 1), male smokers of tobacco had 0.43 mmol/l higher TC levels than male non-smokers. Further, smokers had higher TG levels (especially men), 1.3% higher WHR, and in men, a 4.0 ml/kg/min lower VO_2max than non-smokers. In smokers, the relationship between the amount of tobacco consumption and SBP was modified by gender. In men, a significant positive relationship, and in women a significant negative relationship was found. For every additional cigarette consumed, HDL-C was on average 0.02 mmol/l lower, S4S was 0.1 cm larger, and VO_2max was 0.25 ml/kg/min lower. Changes in the amount of tobacco consumption were significantly and positively related with a TC change in men. Longitudinal analyses on the other CVD risk factors revealed no significant relationships with the 4-year change in the amount of tobacco smoking.

Discussion

Smoking was a risk for all CHD risk factors except BP. This is roughly in line with our hypothesis. Using the change scores of the participants who were their own control revealed hardly any significant relationships (only TC in men) in the regression analyses in spite of the higher statistical power of longitudinal analyses. This absence of significant findings may be caused by the fact that in this group of healthy young adults smoking was a rather stable habit. Between age 32 and 36, not many smokers changed the amount of tobacco smoked and only 20 participants started, while 11 stopped smoking.

Consistent with findings from other studies [14–16] moderate alcohol consumption in the present study is strongly beneficial for HDL-C, even when taking into account the amount of error in the measurement of alcohol consumption and HDL (see paper by Koppes et al. [pp 44–63]). Moderate alcohol use may be as good for DBP in women but not so in men. This result does not correspond to that of Marti's cross-sectional study [16], showing that in both genders, alcohol consumption was associated with elevated levels of SDP and DBP (men: both $p < 0.001$; women: $p = 0.05$ and 0.01, respectively). As for fat distribution (less central) our results are in contrast with other findings [17, 18] and also those of aerobic fitness. With respect to VO_2max, causality may be in the reverse direction. The more fit, the more alcohol was consumed by our subjects, although all of them practiced drinking in moderation. As for other levels of drinking, Kunz [19] showed a curvilinear association between sports participation and the frequency of drinking. Those drinking 2–3 times per week (20–30 years old, regular drinkers) were more active in physical sports than those with a higher or lower drinking frequency. This finding may reflect that sporting and drinking in moderation may belong to a specific lifestyle that is considered as healthy and to which also may belong the level of coffee consumption as found in our group of healthy men and women.

Drinking more coffee only marginally lowered DBP (p = 0.04) which is in line with the inconsistent findings from the vast amount of literature showing either small increases or decreases of blood pressure or no effect. Interesting was that the change in amount of coffee consumption induced a small HDL-C increase. There is hardly any other evidence showing this beneficial effect, although in 10,359 40- to 59-year-old men and women, Brown et al. [20] found that those who did *not* drink coffee had a *higher* prevalence of CHD than coffee drinkers (p < 0.05). Stavric [21] found no relationship between coffee intake and LDL or HDL and a negative association with triglycerides. Jee et al. [22] meta-analyzed 18 intervention studies with healthy subjects on this point and found a dose-response relationship between coffee consumption and TC and LDL (p < 0.01). As for HDL, there was a pooled estimate of 0.2 mg/dl (p = 0.75) increase with a range of −3.9 to 5.0 mg/dl revealing a significant lack of homogeneity (p < 0.0001). Hence, the positive longitudinal HDL-C finding of the present study, although in contrast with the found cross-sectional trend that 0.08 mmol/l lowers HDL-C levels in coffee drinkers as compared with non-drinkers (p = 0.07) might represent a 'true' relationship, although of minor clinical significance. This relationship could be more precise if we had taken into account caffeine intake form other sources than coffee. Also, the level of this unreported intake may depend on the absolute level of coffee consumption. The relative significance of coffee and alcohol use for the HDL-C level is illustrated by our finding showing that the HDL-C effect of a change of four cups of coffee per day (400 mg caffeine) is equivalent to the effect of a change of only 1 alcoholic drink (10 g alcohol).

Globally our findings show that smoking leads to a profile of increased cardiovascular health risk (higher TC, lower HDL-C and lower VO$_2$max levels), while those of alcohol consumption (higher HDL-C, higher dose-dependent VO$_2$max) and coffee consumption (slightly higher HDL-C and lower SBP) show lower risk profiles. Whether non-substance factors, such as motivational or behavioral factors could be at stake is yet not studied in our data, but is an option to consider. Motivational factors in the consumption of these universally accepted products have to do with the ambivalent attitude to these pleasures. With the proverbial pleasure, the relaxation and conviviality these products give, come the feelings of guilt. The relevance of this remark is found in a study by Harburg's group [23]. They searched for the independent contribution of psychosocial variables in predicting hangovers in 1,104 current social drinkers (men: level of alcohol use ranging from <4.2 drinks of 10 g a week to ≥2.8 drinks daily; women: intake range from <4.2 drinks a week to ≥1.4 drink/daily).

By using regression analyses, guilt about drinking formed for both men and women the strongest predictor of hangovers. Since feelings of guilt form a chronic negative stress, and negative stress by its orthosympatic activation is associated with CHD, it may partly explain why to the present day the question on the relationship of smoking, alcohol use and coffee drinking is not answered sufficiently and why relatively more negative health effects are found for smoking than for alcohol use and coffee drinking. From a large survey [24] on smoking came out that 55% of the 4,020 respondents felt guilty about their habit. This figure was 28% for alcohol use and 12% for coffee drinking. Hence, to test whether no smoking and moderate alcohol and coffee consumption are related with healthier levels of the assessed CVD risk factors at first an answer should be given on the influence of psychosocial factors, in particular of positive and negative emotions [25, 26] that go together with the consumption of these pleasure products.

References

1   He J, Vupputuri S, Allen K, Prerost MR, Hughes J, Whelton PK: Passive smoking and the risk of coronary heart disease: A meta-analysis of epidemiologic studies. N Engl J Med 1999;340: 920–926.

2   Ockene IS, Miller NH: Cigarette smoking, cardiovascular disease, and stroke: A statement for healthcare professionals from the American Heart Association. American Heart Association Task Force on Risk Reduction. Circulation 1997;96:3243–3247.

3   Shinton R, Beevers G: Meta-analysis of relation between cigarette smoking and stroke. BMJ 1989;298:789–794.

4   Maclure M: Demonstration of deductive meta-analysis: Ethanol intake and risk of myocardial infarction. Epidemiol Rev 1993;15:328–351.

5   Marmot MG: Alcohol and coronary heart disease. Int J Epidemiol 2001;30:724–729.

6   Corrao G, Rubbiati L, Bagnardi V, Zambon A, Poikolainen K: Alcohol and coronary heart disease: A meta-analysis. Addiction 2000;95:1505–1523.

7   Olson CK, Kutner L, staff of the American Council on Science and Health (ACSH): A Comparison of the Health Effects of Alcohol Consumption and Tobacco Use in America. New York, American Council on Science and Health (ACSH), 2000, pp 1–46. http://www.acsh.org; acsh@acsh.org

8   Kawachi I, Colditz GA, Stone CB: Does coffee drinking increase the risk of coronary heart disease? Results from a meta-analysis. Br Heart J 1994;72:269–275.

9   Greenland S: A meta-analysis of coffee, myocardial infarction, and coronary death. Epidemiology 1993;4:366–374.

10   Nawrot P, Jordan S, Eastwood J, Rotstein J, Hugenholtz A, Feeley M: Effects of caffeine on human health. Food Addit Contam 2003;20:1–30.

11   Lane JD, Pieper CF, Phillips-Bute BG, Bryant JE, Kuhn CM: Caffeine affects cardiovascular and neuroendocrine activation at work and home. Psychosom Med 2002;64:595–603.

12   Grobbee DE, Rimm EB, Giovannucci E, Colditz G, Stampfer M, Willett W: Coffee, caffeine, and cardiovascular disease in men. N Engl J Med 1990;323:1026–1032.

13   Corti R, Binggeli C, Sudano I, Spieker L, Hänseler E, Ruschitzka F, Chaplin WF, Lüscher TF, Noll G: Coffee acutely increases sympathetic nerve activity and blood pressure independently of caffeine content. Circulation 2002;106:2935–2940.

14 Jossa F, Trevisan M, Krogh V, et al: Correlates of high-density lipoprotein cholesterol in a sample of healthy workers. Prev Med 1991;20:700–712.

15 Ellison C: Should physicians prescribe moderate alcohol consumption for the prevention of coronary heart disease? AIM 2000;9:14–15.

16 Marti B, Dai S, Rickenbach M, et al: Total cholesterol, HDL-cholesterol and blood pressure in relation to life style: Results of the first population screening of the Swiss MONIKA Project. Schweiz Med Wochenschr 1990;120:1976–1988.

17 Keil U, Liese A, Filipiak B, Swales JD, Grobbee DE: Alcohol, blood pressure and hypertension. Novartis Found Symp 1998;216:125–144; discussion 144–151.

18 Grobbee DE, Rimm EB, Keil U, Renaud SC: Alcohol and the cardiovascular system; in MacDonald I (ed): Health Issues Related to Alcohol Consumption: ILSI Europe. Oxford, Blackwell Science, 1999, pp 125–179.

19 Kunz JL: Drink and be active? The associations between drinking and participation in sports. Add Res 1997;5:439–450.

20 Brown CA, Bolton-Smith C, Woodward M, Tunstall-Pedoe H: Coffee and tea consumption and the prevalence of coronary heart disease in men and women: Results from the Scottish Heart Health Study. J Epidemiol Community Health 1993;47:171–175.

21 Stavric B: An update on research with coffee/caffeine (1989–1990). Food Chem Toxicol 1992;30:533–555.

22 Jee SH, He J, Appels LJ, Whelton PK, Suh I, Klag MJ: Coffee cosumption and serum lipids: A meta-analysis of randomized controlled clinical trials. Am J Epidemiol 2001;153:353–362.

23 Harburg E, Gunn R, Gleiberman L, Difranceisco W, Schork A: Psychosocial factors, alcohol use and hangover signs among social drinkers: A reappraisal. J Clin Epid 1993;46:413–422.

24 Harris Research Centre: The value of pleasure and the question of guilt – international data tabulations; in Simpson T, Bellchambers L (eds): Research Report JN66029, 1996, p 220.

25 Fredrickson BL, Levenson RW: Positive emotions speed recovery from the cardiovascular sequelae of negative emotions. Cognition Emotion 1998;12:191–220.

26 Perkins K, Grobe JE, Fonte C, Breus M: 'Paradoxical effects' of smoking on subjective stress versus cardiovascular arousal in males and females. Pharmacol Biochem Behav 1992;42:301–311.

Prof. Dr. Han C.G. Kemper
AGAHLS Research Group, Institute for Research in Extramural Medicine
VU University Medical Center,
Van der Boechorststraat 7, NL–1081 BT Amsterdam (The Netherlands)
Tel. +31 20 4448407, Fax +31 20 4446775, E-Mail hcg.kemper.emgo@med.vu.nl

Kemper HCG (ed): Amsterdam Growth and Health Longitudinal Study.
Med Sport Sci. Basel, Karger, 2004, vol 47, pp 132–143

....

Personality, a Determinant of Lifestyle?

Lando L.J. Koppes[a], *Jan Snel*[b], *Han C.G. Kemper*[a]

[a] EMGO Institute, VU University Medical Center, and
[b] Department of Psychology, University of Amsterdam,
Amsterdam, The Netherlands

Abstract

Background/Aims: To investigate the relationships between personality characteristics and lifestyle behaviors. *Methods:* In the participants of the Amsterdam Growth and Health Longitudinal Study, the Dutch Personality Inventory (DPI) and lifestyle behaviors were assessed at ages 32 and 36 years. Cross-sectional and longitudinal regression analyses were performed with the seven DPI sub-scales (Inadequacy, Social Inadequacy, Rigidity, Hostility, Self-sufficiency, Dominance, and Self-esteem) as determinants of five lifestyle behaviors (alcohol, coffee, and tobacco consumption, physical activity, and dietary saturated fat intake). *Results:* Each personality characteristic was found significantly related with at least one of the lifestyle behaviors. Most of the significant results were found in the cross-sectional analyses. *Conclusion:* Whether or not the different lifestyle behaviors are related to a particular single personality profile remains unclear. However, a trend was seen for more healthy lifestyles in the men and women with a more 'easy-going' personality.

Characteristics of an unhealthy lifestyle such as too little physical activity, smoking, irregular and unbalanced diet, over-consumption of alcohol and coffee are assumed to have relationships with major health problems like cardiovascular disease, cancer, and osteoporosis. One of the first signs of impaired health are sleep problems. Fabsitz et al. [1] showed that age, non-participation in group activities, a lack of social support, and lifestyle variables were associated with higher risks to sleep problems. Obviously, a change of unhealthy lifestyle behaviors to more healthy levels will have a large positive impact on public health, and even more so when considered over a period of decades.

It also known that in spite of intensive efforts, lifestyle changes and especially long-term changes appear hard to achieve. It might be that lifestyle behaviors are this stable because they follow a person's personality [2]. The observation of clustering of unhealthy lifestyles [3] may also be the result of this uniform personality underlying unhealthy lifestyles.

Some studies have found relationships between personality characteristics and the occurrence of health problems, but this relationship remains controversial [4, 5]. The classic research of personality as expressed in characteristic illness-related behavior patterns was done by Friedman and Rosenman [6]. They made plausible that an aggressive, impatient, time-urgent and hostile pattern of behavior made people, especially men, prone to coronary heart disease. Another behavior pattern is the cancer-prone behavioral type. Persons with the so-called C-type behavior are overly cooperative, unassertive, avoiding conflict, extremely compliant and are unable to deal with stress which may altogether lead to hopelessness/helplessness or even depression [7].

Since behavior patterns may originate from the individual's personality a more straightforward approach to untwine the presumed association of personality and health is to focus on personality characteristics itself. Indeed, personality characteristics have been found to be related to different lifestyle behaviors. For example, people who score high on novelty or sensation seeking, or extraversion have been found to indulge in eating sweets [8], drinking alcohol [9, 10] or coffee [11, 12], and smoking [13].

In this chapter, the relationships between seven personality characteristics and five lifestyle behaviors are investigated. Moderate consumption of alcohol and coffee, no tobacco, a high level of physical activity, and a low percentage of energy intake from saturated fat were considered to be the healthy lifestyle behaviors. If a single personality profile is found that predicts the cluster of unhealthy lifestyle behaviors, an explanation is found for the clustering of unhealthy lifestyle behaviors, and for the difficulty to achieve lasting lifestyle improvements. More importantly, knowledge of such a single personality profile that underlies unhealthy lifestyle behaviors may be of great help in the development of lifestyle interventions that work better and last longer.

Methods

Personality Characteristics
Personality characteristics were assessed using the Dutch Personality Inventory (DPI) [14, 15]. The DPI includes the following scales:
1   Inadequacy (IN): vague feelings of malfunctioning, anxiety, vague physical and psychosomatic complaints, depressive mood;

---

2   Social Inadequacy (SI): neurotic shyness, uncomfortable feelings in social situations, avoidance of unfamiliar people or situations;

3   Rigidity (RG): the need for regularity, having fixed habits and principles, sense of duty and a positive task appraisal, perseverance;

4   Hostility (HO): mistrust, intolerance, impatience;

5   Self-sufficiency or recalcitrance (SS): desire to solve problems alone, feelings of independence;

6   Dominance (DO): self-reliance, trying to be or play the boss;

7   Self-esteem (SE): concurrence between actual and preferred daily pursuits and self-image, optimism, vitality.

    The construction of the DPI was based on the California Psychological Inventory [16].

Lifestyle Behaviors

The lifestyle behaviors studied in this chapter are physical activity (MET/week), smoking (cigarettes/day), alcohol (glasses/day) and coffee consumption (cups/day), and the percentage of total dietary energy intake in the form of saturated fat. Physical activity was assessed using a face-to-face interview, and was calculated as the metabolic intensity of performed activities times the duration of those activities [17]. Activities of less than 4 times the basal metabolic rate (<4 METs) were not taken into account. Tobacco smoking and coffee consumption were assessed using a questionnaire, while alcohol consumption and dietary energy intake were assessed using a face-to-face interview that included crosschecks [18].

Analyses

The data obtained at age 32 years were investigated on the cross-sectional relationships between 5-point differences on the DPI sub-scales and consuming or not consuming tobacco, alcohol or coffee. These logistic regression analyses resulted in odds ratios (ORs) which indicate that a 5-point higher score on a personality sub-scale is related to an OR times higher chance to be a consumer. In consumers, linear regression analyses were performed with the amount of tobacco smoking, alcohol and coffee consumption at age 32 years as dependent variables. These linear analyses were performed also with regard to the amount of physical activity, and the percentage of dietary energy intake from saturated fat. Because these lifestyle data were skewed to the right, the natural logarithm of these variables was used. These second analyses indicate that a 5-point higher score on a personality characteristic is related to an exp(b) times higher score on the lifestyle habit. Thus, in the relationship between personality characteristics and lifestyle behaviors, an exp(b) is indicative for the level of the lifestyle behavior in an equivalent way as an OR is indicative for the chance to consume or to abstain from tobacco, alcohol, or coffee.

Next to these cross-sectional analyses, longitudinal analyses were performed using the changes between ages 32 and 36 years of all variables of interest. These change-scores were calculated by subtracting the value obtained at age 36 from the value obtained at age 32 years. Because the change scores of the lifestyle behaviors were not skewed, log-transformation was not needed here, and the results of the regression analyses indicate the relationship between a 5-point increase on a personality characteristic and the absolute change on the lifestyle behavior.

Interactions between personality characteristics and gender are analyzed, and if significant, stratified analyses are performed, and if not significant, analyses are controlled for gender.

Table 1. Means (SD) of the personality characteristics at age 32 years, and the changes observed over the following 4 years

	Men		Women	
	age 32	change	age 32	change
Inadequacy	7.1 (5.8)	−0.8 (4.9)	9.4 (6.2)	−0.1 (5.6)
Social Inadequacy	7.0 (6.4)	−0.6 (3.9)	8.8 (7.1)	−0.2 (4.2)
Rigidity	21.3 (6.8)	0.1 (5.2)	23.1 (6.9)	0.9 (5.0)
Hostility	13.1 (6.6)	−0.4 (4.4)	13.6 (6.4)	−0.3 (4.5)
Self-Sufficiency	10.6 (4.7)	−0.5 (4.1)	8.4 (4.0)	−0.0 (3.1)
Dominance	19.0 (6.4)	0.2 (4.2)	15.2 (6.2)	0.3 (4.0)
Self-Esteem	30.5 (5.9)	0.2 (4.4)	29.8 (4.8)	−0.8 (4.0)

Table 2. Percentages, means (SD) of the lifestyle behaviors at age 32 years, and the changes observed over the following 4 years

		Men		Women	
		age 32	change	age 32	change
Alcohol	% drinker	89	1	73	1
	g/drinker/day	16.0 (17.6)	3.4 (13.0)	9.0 (11.3)	5.7 (14.3)
Coffee	% drinker	77	15	77	9
	cups/drinker/day	4.8 (4.0)	0.8 (2.8)	3.6 (3.0)	0.2 (2.0)
Tobacco	% smoker	26	1	19	1
	g/smoker/day	10.5 (9.7)	0.5 (9.3)	12.4 (7.9)	−0.0 (9.3)
Physical activity	kMET/week	3.3 (2.3)	1.2 (2.6)	3.5 (2.4)	1.8 (3.5)
Saturated fat	% energy intake	14.1 (2.8)	−0.6 (2.5)	14.8 (2.8)	−0.9 (3.1)

Results

Descriptive data of the personality characteristics are shown in table 1. As compared with a representative Dutch norm-group [14] the AGAHLS participants at the age of 32 years had average to below average IN, SI, RG, HO, and SS, average to above average DO, and average SE. The average changes on the DPI sub-scale scores between ages 32 and 36 were small, while the SD's of these changes were relatively large given the presumption that personality characteristics are relatively stable.

In table 2, descriptive data of the lifestyle behaviors are shown. Most AGAHLS men and women appeared to be moderate drinkers, but the amount

Table 3. Odds ratios (ORs) and 95% CI regarding relationships between a 5 point difference in DPI sub-scales and consuming or not consuming alcohol, coffee or tobacco at age 32 years

	Alcohol		Coffee		Tobacco	
	OR	95% CI	OR	95% CI	OR	95% CI
Inadequacy	0.92	0.76–1.11	1.11	0.92–1.35	1.13	0.94–1.36
Social Inadequacy	0.84	0.70–0.99	1.02	0.86–1.20	0.92	0.77–1.10
Rigidity	M 0.98	0.71–1.35	0.99	0.84–1.17	0.85	0.72–1.02
	W 0.58	0.45–0.73				
Hostility	0.81	0.67–0.97	M 0.80	0.62–1.04	1.03	0.86–1.24
			W 1.19	0.93–1.52		
Self-Sufficiency	0.68	0.51–0.91	1.07	0.82–1.39	M 1.23	0.88–1.73
					W 0.62	0.39–0.98
Dominance	1.03	0.85–1.26	1.06	0.89–1.27	1.10	0.91–1.32
Self-Esteem	0.91	0.71–1.17	0.98	0.79–1.22	0.75	0.61–0.92

of alcohol consumed increased. At age 32 years, 77% of the men and women were consumers of coffee. These male and female drinkers consumed an average of 4.8 and 3.6 cups per day, respectively. Over the following 4 years, this percentage of coffee drinkers showed a strong increase (15% in men, and 9% in women). The amount of coffee per drinker increased as well, with 0.8 cups per day in men, and with 0.2 cups per day in women. About 1 in every 4 men, and 1 in every 5 women reported to smoke tobacco. A change in assessment method has probably caused most of the increase in the level of physical activity in both men and women. At age 32 years, the percentage of the total energy intake in the form of saturated fat was higher in women than in men (14.8 and 14.1%, respectively). These percentages are higher than advised by the health council of the Netherlands, which advises a maximum of 10% [19]. The relative contribution of saturated fat in total energy intake changed towards healthier values over the following 4 years. An average decrease of 0.6% in men, and 0.9% in women was seen.

The results of the logistic regression analyses on the relationships between the DPI sub-scales and the consumption or abstention of alcohol, coffee and tobacco are shown in table 3. Five-point differences in the DPI sub-scales are used in the analyses as the unit of the dependent variables. To get an idea about the magnitude of this unit, the reader is referred to compare the five points with the standard deviations of the personality characteristics that are given in table 1. At age 32, the DPI sub-scales Inadequacy and Dominance were not related with the consumption or abstention of alcohol, coffee or tobacco. A 5-point higher score on Social Inadequacy, Hostility, Self-Sufficiency, and, in women, Rigidity was related with smaller chances to be an alcohol consumer (16, 19, 32 and 42%, respectively). None of the personality characteristics were significantly related with the consumption or abstention of coffee. With respect to the consumption of tobacco, a 5-point higher score on Self-Esteem, and, in women, on Self-Sufficiency was related with a 25 and 38% smaller chance to be a smoker, respectively.

The interpretation of the exp(b)s in table 4 is comparable to that of the ORs in table 3, except, the exp(b)s are based on the lifestyle behaviors as continuous variables. In table 4, the results do not refer to consuming or not, but to the amount of alcohol, coffee and tobacco consumed by those who do drink or smoke, and analogously, to the level of physical activity, respectively, the relative contribution of saturated fat in dietary energy intake.

In men, a 5-point higher score on the DPI sub-scale Inadequacy was related with a 16% higher amount of alcohol consumption. Women who scored 5 points higher on Social Inadequacy, on average, consumed 15% less alcohol, 9% less coffee, and were 10% less active, while women who scored 5 points higher on Rigidity had a slightly higher relative intake of saturated fat. Hostility and Self-Sufficiency were not significantly related with the levels of the lifestyle behaviors, whereas a 5 point higher score on Dominance was related with a 22% smaller amount of tobacco smoking. Finally, a 5 point higher score on Self-Esteem was related with 26% more alcohol consumption and with an 8% higher level of physical activity.

In table 5, the results of the linear regression analyses on the change scores are presented. Only two relationships were found statistically significant. An increase of 5 points on the DPI sub-scale Dominance was related with an increase of about half a cup of coffee per day (0.42), and such an increase on the sub-scale Self-Esteem was related with a decrease in the amount of tobacco smoking of almost one (0.78) cigarette per day.

Discussion

In this chapter, an attempt was made to discern one personality profile as a determinant of several health-related lifestyle behaviors. Several significant results were found for the separate DPI sub-scales. A high score on Inadequacy and Social Inadequacy was negatively related to coffee consumption, while Social Inadequacy was negatively related to coffee and alcohol consumption, and physical activity. The DPI sub-scale Rigidity showed negative relationships with alcohol and tobacco consumption, and a positive relationship with

Table 4. Exp[b]'s and 95% CI's regarding relationships between a 5 point difference on DPI sub-scales and the level of alcohol, coffee or tobacco consumption, physical activity and energy intake at the age of 32 years

	Alcohol		Coffee		Tobacco		Physical activity		Saturated fat	
	Exp[b]	95% CI	Exp[b]	95% CI	Exp[b]	95% CI	Exp[b]	95% CI	Exp[b]	95% CI
Inadequacy	M 1.16 W 0.89	1.02–1.31 0.77–1.03	M 1.09 W 0.93	0.99–1.20 0.87–1.00	1.09	0.92–1.30	M 1.05 W 0.94	0.96–1.15 0.88–1.00	1.00	0.99–1.02
Social Inadequacy	M 1.01 W 0.85	0.90–1.13 0.74–0.96	M 1.05 W 0.91	0.96–1.14 0.86–0.96	1.13	0.94–1.36	M 1.00 W 0.90	0.92–1.09 0.85–0.96	1.01	0.99–1.02
Rigidity	0.94	0.86–1.02	M 1.05 W 0.95	0.97–1.14 0.90–1.01	0.91	0.77–1.08	0.98	0.93–1.02	M 0.99 W 1.02	0.96–1.01 1.00–1.04
Hostility	0.97	0.88–1.06	M 1.05 W 0.94	0.97–1.14 0.88–1.00	0.94	0.78–1.14	1.03	0.98–1.08	0.99	0.98–1.01
Self-Sufficiency	0.90	0.79–1.03	0.97	0.90–1.05	0.84	0.66–1.06	1.04	0.96–1.12	1.00	0.98–1.03
Dominance	1.00	0.89–1.12	1.02	0.97–1.08	0.78	0.66–0.92	1.04	0.99–1.10	1.00	0.99–1.02
Self-Esteem	1.26	1.09–1.45	1.01	0.95–1.08	0.91	0.76–1.09	1.08	1.01–1.15	1.00	0.98–1.02

Table 5. Regression coefficients and 95% CI's regarding relationships between a 5 point change on DPI sub-scales and the change of alcohol, coffee or tobacco consumption, physical activity and percentage energy intake from saturated fat between the age of 32 and 36 years

	Alcohol (glass/day)		Coffee (cup/day)		Tobacco (cigarette/day)		Physical activity (MET/week)		Saturated fat (% of energy intake)	
	b	95% CI	b	95% CI	b	95% CI	b	95% CI	b	95% CI
Inadequacy	-0.03	-0.14–0.09	-0.08	-0.32–0.16	0.02	-0.37–0.40	61	-254–376	0.26	-0.03–0.55
Social Inadequacy	-0.04	-0.19–0.11	-0.08	-0.39–0.23	-0.12	-0.63–0.39	46	-364–456	0.23	-0.14–0.61
Rigidity	-0.10	-0.22–0.02	-0.18	-0.43–0.07	-0.17	-0.57–0.24	-71	-400–259	0.15	-0.16–0.45
Hostility	0.02	-0.11–0.15	0.12	-0.17–0.41	0.25	-0.22–0.72	40	-334–414	0.20	-0.15–0.54
Self-Sufficiency	-0.05	-0.22–0.12	0.25	-0.12–0.62	0.21	-0.39–0.81	-359	-823–105	0.13	-0.30–0.56
Dominance	-0.11	-0.25–0.04	0.42	0.11–0.74	-0.05	-0.56–0.46	-252	-656–151	0.14	-0.23–0.52
Self-Esteem	-0.08	-0.22–0.06	0.14	-0.16–0.45	-0.78	-1.27 to -0.29	-151	-548–246	-0.09	-0.45–0.27

saturated fat intake. A more hostile personality appeared related to less alcohol and coffee consumption, while the participants who scored higher on Self-Sufficiency more often abstained from alcohol or tobacco, or drank less coffee. The more dominant participants less likely were firm tobacco smokers, while those who increased on Dominance also increased on coffee consumption. Finally, the score on the DPI sub-scale Self-Esteem was negatively related to smoking tobacco, and positively related to the amount of alcohol consumption and physical activity. Overall there appears to be a trend for healthier lifestyle behaviors in those with a more easy-going personality (i.e. low (Social) Inadequacy, Rigidity, Hostility, and Self-Sufficiency, and high Dominance and Self-Esteem).

In a way, this observed trend of a single profile, constructed from several personality sub-scales is not very plausible from a theoretical point of view. Per definition, personality is considered as consisting of statistically independent factors. The same is true for lifestyle factors as found by Vingerhoets et al. [20]. They defined as a positive lifestyle: 7–8 h of sleep per day, breakfasting almost every day, rarely eating snacks between meals, being at or near prescribed body-weight, never smoking, moderate or no use of alcohol and regular physical activity. The inter-correlations moved around 0.10, with the highest being 0.20 between breakfasting and smoking and smoking and alcohol. Such low correlations are typical for consumption habits as was demonstrated in an extensive review [21]. Use of recreational substances may belong to one underlying factor as was indicated by factor analytical results showing that the consumption of alcohol (factor loading 0.57), coffee (factor loading 0.52) and smoking (factor loading 0.82) belong to one factor. Except for using such inter-correlated habits in general, lifestyle is still a weak heterogeneous construct. Using such a concept together with orthogonally related personality traits in order to find a specific personality profile to explain lifestyle certainly is difficult.

The above-outlined difficulty could explain our relatively few statistically significant findings on the longitudinal analyses. A relationship between an increase in Dominance and the amount of coffee consumption, and a relationship between an increase in Self-Esteem with a decrease in the amount of tobacco smoked, were the only two significant longitudinal findings. Another explanation could be the relatively high stability of the variables involved, because if personality or lifestyle behaviors would hardly change over the four years of follow-up, this would inevitably result in low statistical power of the longitudinal analyses. This was not the case for the lifestyle behaviors, as is outlined in chapter 5. However, the partial inter-period correlation coefficients of the personality characteristics between the ages of 32 and 36 years were relatively high, with values between 0.65 and 0.81. A third explanation could be that the cross-sectional relationships that are found statistically significant do not represent a causal association between personality and lifestyle behaviors, but that their association is caused by a third underlying factor. For example, persons raised in a very conservative, or urban, or religious environment may report different on both personality and lifestyle questions than those raised in a more liberal or rural environment. Confounding therefore may have caused the found significant relationships.

Another comment could be given on the selected behavioral characteristics that should form lifestyle. Almost exclusively, lifestyle is based on conceptions of good or bad health. Views on healthy lifestyle behaviors however vary among researchers depending on bias, see for example for coffee consumption [22, 23] and on culture as has been shown for alcohol [24]. The latter author showed that the amount of alcohol consumption at which all-cause mortality is least is in the USA 6.9 units per week, while in the UK it is 11.6. Due to these diverging views on which habits are contributing to good health or are harmful, it will be no surprise that attempts to link personality to lifestyle will easily result in different findings between studies. Neither, there is consensus with regard to the level of consumption of substances or food products that is presumed healthy or harmful. Even health organizations have different opinions on what is safe to health. For example, despite the ample evidence showing that alcohol consumed in moderate amounts is contributing consistently to good health [25, 26], some studies consider any alcohol as harmful. Not unexpected in this respect, opinions on what is good for health may change in the course of time as well [27, 28].

In spite of these comments, the results of the present analyses do confirm what is found in general in the literature. Sensation, or novelty seeking, and extraversion go together with risk taking behavior such as not wearing safety belts and consummatory, indulgent behavior that could be indicative of a certain risk to health. Also, adherence to a prudent, healthy lifestyle (not drinking alcohol, not smoking, a regular sleep and having meals, no snacks, exercising regularly, and taking a well-balanced diet with sufficient fruit and dairy products) as reflected in a strict compliance to guidelines, may result from social insecurity and introversion. An intriguing way to explain why differences in lifestyle are based on personality results from the idea that personality is determined from a common underlying physiological activation or arousal level. Arousal level might be the common factor [29] that underlies personality traits as extraversion-introversion, impulsiveness and sensation seeking. This assumption based on the theories of Eysenck [29] and Revelle [30] implies that under identical conditions introverts are physiologically more highly aroused than extraverts, low impulsives more than high impulsives, and low sensation seekers more than high sensation seekers, and by that are inclined to a lifestyle that is less challenging and risky than that of extraverts and (socially) secure people. In other words the more highly aroused persons may tend to lower consumption levels of 'risky' substances as caffeine, alcohol, nicotine and may be less sporting and outgoing types and thus have a more prudent and an assumed more healthy lifestyle than extraverted, high sensations seekers. The validity of this hypothesis that a higher or more stable level of arousal underlies the more 'easy-going' personality that appears to be related with healthier lifestyle behaviors is a matter of future analyses.

References

1 Fabsitz RR, Sholinsky P, Goldberg J: Correlates of sleep problems among men: The Vietnam Era Twin Registry. J Sleep Res 1997;6:50–56.
2 Mehrabian A: Pleasure-arousal-dominance: A general framework for describing and measuring individual differences in temperament. Current Psychology 1996;14:261–292.
3 Twisk JWR, Kemper HCG, van Mechelen W, Post GB: Clustering of risk factors for coronary heart disease: The longitudinal relationship with lifestyle. Ann Epidemiol 2001;11:157–165.
4 Butow PN, Hiller JE, Price MA, Thackway SV, Kricker A, Tennant CC: Epidemiological evidence for a relationship between life events, coping style, and personality factors in the development of breast cancer. J Psychosom Res 2000;49:169–181.
5 Myrtek M: Meta-analyses of prospective studies on coronary heart disease, type A personality, and hostility. Int J Cardiol 2001;79:245–251.
6 Friedman S, Rosenman RH: Type A Behavior and Your Heart. New York, Knops, 1974.
7 Eysenck HJ: Personality, stress and cancer: Prediction and prophylaxis. Br J Med Psychol 1988; 61:57–75.
8 Rozin P, Stoess C: Is there a general tendency to become addicted? Addict Behav 1993;18:81–87.
9 Andrew M, Cronin C: Two measures of sensations seeking as predictors of alcohol use among high school males. Person Ind Diff 1997;22:393–401.
10 Grau E, Ortet G: Personality traits and alcohol consumption in a sample of non-alcoholic women. Pers Indiv Diff 1999;27:1057–1066.
11 Andrucci GL, Archer RP, Pancoast DL, Gordon RA: The relationship of MMPI and Sensation Seeking Scales to adolescent drug use. J Pers Assess 1989;53:253–266.
12 Brice CF, Smith AP: Factors associated with caffeine consumption. Int J Food Sci Nutr 2002;53: 55–64.
13 Pritchard WS, Robinson JH, deBethizy JD, Davis RA, Stiles MF: Caffeine and smoking: Subjective, performance, and psychophysiological effects. Psychophysiology 1995;32:19–27.
14 Luteijn F, Starren J, Van Dijk H: Manual for the Dutch Personality Inventory (in Dutch). Lisse, Swets en Zeitlinger b.v., 1985.
15 Luteijn F: The Construction of a Personality Inventory (in Dutch). Groningen, Rijksuniversiteit Groningen, 1974.
16 Gough HG: Manual for the California Psychological Inventory. Palo Alto, Consulting Psychological Inventory, 1964.
17 Montoye HJ, Kemper HCG, Saris WHM, Washburn RA: Measuring Physical Activity and Energy Expenditure. Champaign, Human Kinetics, 1996.
18 Bakker I, Twisk JW, Van Mechelen W, Mensink GB, Kemper HC: Computerization of a dietary history interview in a running cohort: Evaluation within the Amsterdam Growth and Health Longitudinal Study. Eur J Clin Nutr 2003;57:394–404.
19 Health Council of the Netherlands, Committee on Trends in Food Consumption (Gezondheidsraad): Significant Trends in Food Consumption in the Netherlands (in Dutch). The Hague, Health Council of the Netherlands, 2002.
20 Vingerhoets AJJM, Croon M, Jeninga AJ, Menges LJ: Personality and health habits. Psychol Hlth 1990;4:333–342.

21   Istvan J, Matarazzo JD: Tobacco, alcohol, and caffeine use: A review of their interrelationships. Psychol Bull 1984;95:301–326.

22   James JE: Caffeine, health and commercial interests. Addiction 1994;89:1595–1599.

23   Jee SH, He J, Appel LJ, Whelton PK, Suh I, Klag MJ: Coffee consumption and serum lipids: A meta-analysis of randomized controlled clinical trials. Am J Epidemiol 2001;153:353–362.

24   White IR: The level of alcohol consumption at which all-cause mortality is least. J Clin Epidemiol 1999;52:967–975.

25   Koppes LL, Twisk JW, Snel J, Van Mechelen W, Kemper HC: Blood cholesterol levels of 32-year-old alcohol consumers are better than of nonconsumers. Pharmacol Biochem Behav 2000;66: 163–167.

26   Snel J: A drink, a healthy pleasure. Alcohol Moderation 2002;11:17.

27   Gorman C: Walk, don't run. Time 2002;159:54–56.

28   Horowitz JM: 10 Foods that pack a wallop – Eat, drink and be healthy. Time 2002;159:48–53.

29   Bullock WA, Gilliland K: Eysenck's arousal theory of introversion-extraversion: A converging measures investigation. J Pers Soc Psychol 1993;64:113–123.

30   Revelle W, Humphreys MS, Simon L, Gilliland K: The interactive effect of personality, time of day, and caffeine: A test of the arousal model. J Exp Psychol Gen 1980;109:1–31.

Prof. Dr. Han C.G. Kemper
AGAHLS Research Group, Institute for Research in Extramural Medicine
VU University Medical Center
Van der Boechorststraat 7, NL–1081 BT Amsterdam (The Netherlands)
Tel. +31 20 4448407, Fax +31 20 4446775, E-Mail hcg.kemper.emgo@med.vu.nl

Kemper HCG (ed): Amsterdam Growth and Health Longitudinal Study.
Med Sport Sci. Basel, Karger, 2004, vol 47, pp 144–152

....

Energy Balance in Relation to Body Composition from Adolescence to Adulthood

Han C.G. Kemper, Lando L.J. Koppes

Institute for Research in Extramural Medicine (EMGO Institute),
VU University Medical Center (VUmc), Amsterdam, The Netherlands

Abstract

Background/Aims: The alarming increase in the prevalence of obesity demands for information on the relationships of dietary intake (DI) and physical activity (PA) with the development of fat mass. *Methods:* Data from eight repeated measurements from age 13 through 36 years in 698 subjects from the Amsterdam Growth And Health Longitudinal Study (AGAHLS) were used to analyze the relationships of actual values and changes of PA and DI with body mass index (BMI) and the sum of four skinfolds (S4S). *Results:* Regression analyses using generalized estimating equations showed that a 1 SD higher PA was related with a $0.18 \, kg/m^2$ smaller BMI and a $0.10 \, cm$ smaller S4S in men. In women no significant relationships were found. Unexpectedly, lower DI values were related with a higher S4S and (in women) BMI. Underreporting of DI was the probable cause of these negative relationships, because analyses on DI changes showed no relationships with body composition. **Conclusion:** PA in males is negatively related and DI is not related with BMI and S4S. Therefore, promotion of physical activity may be more effective in the prevention of obesity.

Since the 1960s there has been a clear increase in the prevalence of over-weightness (BMI >25) and obesity (BMI >30) not only in the US and Canada [1] but also in Europe. In the Netherlands the prevalence of obesity was estimated in 1997 to be as high as 7% for adult men and 11% for adult women [2]. The increase is discernable in youth also [3]. Moreover there seems to be a clear relation between obesity and other biological risk indicators of cardiovascular diseases [4] such as hypertension, hypercholesterolemia and type II diabetes. Obesity during childhood and adolescence is supposed to be an important determinant of whether a subject will become obese as an adult [5–7]. It has been found that 40% of children who were obese at age 7 years became obese adults, whereas more than 70% of obese adolescents became obese adults [7].

Apart from genetic and environmental factors [8] also lifestyle factors are associated with the development of obesity in youth. Important lifestyles in this respect are physical activity, dietary intake and early events in fetal and infantile growth. Food follows activity and the regulation of the energy balance and body weight seems to function better in situations where the demand of energy output is high and the energy intake is low. In modern western societies the situation is reversed (high energy intake and low energy output), leading to a gradual increase in body weight. Most prevention programs are focussed on healthy diets and a more physically active life because these two lifestyles are thought to be of major importance in the development of obesity. Therefore, successful prevention of obesity may need to be started as early as in the growing years of the adolescence and should probably be focused on dietary habits and habitual physical activity. This chapter concerns the longitudinal relationship of dietary intake and physical activity with two body composition measures (BMI and the Sum of Four Skinfolds) in a group of 13-year-old healthy boys and girls, that are followed over a period of 23 years till the age of 36 years, as part of the Amsterdam Growth And Health Longitudinal Study (AGAHLS) [9, 10].

Methods

The Amsterdam Growth And Health Longitudinal Study (AGAHLS) used a multiple longitudinal design with repeated measurements in three birth cohorts (1962, 1963 and 1964) of males and females. The subjects were recruited as a whole sample from two secondary schools in Amsterdam and Purmerend (The Netherlands). Between 1976 and 2000 eight repeated measurements are completed: during the school period (13–16 years) four annual measurements, a fifth in 1985 (mean age 21 years), a sixth in 1991 (mean age 27 years), a seventh in 1996/1997 (mean age 32 years), and an eighth measurement in 2000 (mean age 36 years). Over the 23-year period the total drop-out rate was about 35%. For the analyses in this study, data were used from all 698 participants (331 men and 367 women) who on average attended 3.65 of the eight measurements.

The method to measure anthropometric and lifestyle factors have not changed over the 23 years of follow-up. All eight measurements were performed with identical procedures in all subjects. Anthropometric measurements of body height, body mass and four skinfolds (biceps, triceps, subscapular and crista iliac) were performed according standard procedures [11]. Body mass index (BMI), the ratio between body mass (kg) and body height squared (m^2), was used as an indirect measure of fat mass. The sum of four skinfolds (S4S) was used as a more direct measure of fat mass [12].

Two lifestyle factors have been monitored, dietary intake (DI), and physical activity (PA). DI was measured with a modification of the crosscheck dietary history interview that referred to the last month [13]. All subjects were interviewed by a dietitian to recall their usual intake of foods and drinks by reporting (a) the frequency (limited to at least twice a month); (b) the amounts (with models used to illustrate common portion sizes such as glasses, bowls, spoons and imitations of sizes of potatoes and fruits; a pair of scales to weigh sugar and butter addition), and (c) methods of preparation of the foods consumed. All consumed food items were transformed into nutrients in accordance with the Dutch Food and Nutrition Table [14]. As parameter of DI is chosen for the total energy intake (MJ/day).

Physical activity was measured with a standardized cross-check activity interview that was based on a questionnaire [15]. The interview was retrospective over the previous 3 months and covered the following areas: organized sports activities, unorganized sports activities (e.g. playing in the street), active transportation (e.g. bicycling), activities at home (gardening, playing with children), school (physical education) and at work (stair climbing). Only those physical activities were taken into account with a minimal duration of 5 min and an intensity level of four times basal metabolic rate (4 Mets). The physical activities were classified in three intensity levels: 4–7, 7–10, and >10 Mets, respectively [16]. The PA score was calculated as the average weekly time (minutes) spent, multiplied by the respective level of intensity. This weighted energy expenditure (Met · min/week) was used as the PA score for each year of measurement. In the last measurement period (2000) DI and PA were measured with a computerized version of the interviews [17].

Linear regression analyses were performed with Generalized Estimating Equations to study the relationship of DI and PA with BMI and S4S [18, 19]. To avoid that the longitudinal development of DI and PA confound the relationship with S4S and BMI, gender-specific z-scores of DI and PA were used. Analyses were performed both with actual values and with delta values (time n minus time n–1), and corrections were made for gender and age. In the analyses PA was corrected for DI and vice versa.

Results

In table 1 means and standard deviations of the variables used in this study are summarized for the male and female participants at the eighth measurement at the mean age of 36 years. The differences between sexes are statistically significant in all anthropometric measures ($p < 0.01$). Males show significantly higher DI and lower PA than females.

The longitudinal results of DI between age 13 and 36 years showed an increase in energy intake in males from about 11.3 MJ per day at age 13 years to about 13.3 MJ per day at age 21 years, followed by a slight decrease to 12.5 MJ per day at age 36 years. In females the mean energy intake hardly changed between 13 and 36 years of age with mean values between 8.9 and 9.7 MJ per day. Males showed significantly higher energy intakes than females, at each year of measurement.

The longitudinal results of PA showed a steep decrease in the energy expenditure in both sexes from age 13 to age 16: in boys from about 4,700 Mets per week to about 3,700 Mets per week and in girls from 3,800 to 3,200 Mets per week

Table 1. Means and SD of subject characteristics at the mean age of 36 years

	Males (n = 178)		Females (n = 200)	
Age, years	36.0	(0.8)	36.1	(0.7)
Body height, cm	184	(6)	170	(6)
Body mass, kg	83.8	(10.7)	67.9	(10.2)
S4S, mm	47	(15)	55	(19)
BMI, kg/m^2	24.8	(2.7)	23.4	(3.3)
DI, MJ/day	12.5	(3.1)	9.7	(2.1)
PA, kMET/week	4.4	(2.7)	5.4	(3.7)

S4S = Sum of four skinfolds; BMI = body mass index; PA = physical activity; DI = dietary intake.

(see chapter by Kemper and Koppes [pp 158–159]). During adolescence, boys showed a 20% higher energy expenditure than girls. From the age of 21 to 32 years, PA stabilized at mean values between 2,900 and 3,600 Mets per week and there were no distinct differences between males and females. At age 36 years, when the computerized assessment method was used, PA was increased in both sexes and the females showed mean values of 5,400 Mets per week compared to males with 4,400 Mets per week.

The longitudinal relationship of the actual values of PA with BMI and S4S (table 2) resulted in significant (p = 0.02) negative regression coefficients in males but not in females. These regression coefficients should be interpreted as the following example: a one SD higher PA score was related to a 0.18 kg/m^2 higher BMI and a 0.10 cm smaller S4S. With DI however, the regression coefficients with S4S were significant in males and females and with BMI only in females, but these were not in the expected direction: one SD lower DI in males and females respectively, was related with 0.10 cm and 0.23 cm higher S4S and only in females related with a 0.16 kg/m^2 higher BMI.

Using the delta scores, an increase in PA was related with decreases in S4S and BMI, but only significant for S4S in males. The delta values of DI were not related with S4S and BMI changes.

Discussion

We found indeed that higher S4S and BMI values were related with a lower PA, but surprisingly also with lower DI. This unexpected result that a 23 years

Table 2. Regression coefficients (mean and 95% CI) of actual and delta values of dietary intake (DI, z-scores), and physical activity (PA, z-scores) with sum of four skinfolds (S4S, cm) and Body Mass Index (BMI, kg/m^2) of males and females over a period of 23 years between age 13 and 36 years

			Actual values		Change scores	
			b	95% CI	b	95% CI
PA	Men	S4S	−0.10	−0.19; −0.02	−0.06	−0.12; 0.00
		BMI	−0.18	−0.33; −0.03	−0.07	−0.17; 0.03
	Women	S4S	−0.04	−0.12; 0.05	−0.06	−0.14; 0.02
		BMI	0.06	−0.07; 0.19	−0.04	−0.14; 0.07
DI	Men	S4S	−0.10	−0.18; −0.03	−0.05	−0.12; 0.02
		BMI	0.10	−0.04; 0.24	0.06	−0.05; 0.17
	Women	S4S	−0.23	−0.33; −0.14	0.01	−0.09; 0.10
		BMI	−0.16	−0.30; −0.03	0.09	−0.03; 0.21

lower energy intake is related to a higher fat mass can be explained in two ways: (1) Well known is the phenomenon of underreporting of DI: overweight and obese subjects are prone to 'forget' food stuffs or foodstuffs with a high energy density consumed in order to please the interviewer. Goris et al. [20] found in obese patients a 30% underreporting of foodstuffs with a high fat percentage. (2) Repeated measurements, as in this longitudinal study can introduce negative testing effects as was found in the boys during adolescence [21]. That systematic differential underreporting could be the case is proved by the fact that analyses with delta values of DI with S4S and BMI resulted in coefficients that indicate positive trends.

During adolescence and young adulthood in the population of males and females from the AGAHLS the PA decreased rapidly, but the DI, increased in males during adolescence but not in females. DI and PA stabilized in both sexes between 21 and 36 years.

Fat mass, indirectly measured from BMI and S4S, increased gradually in both sexes between 13 and 36 years. This development resulted in an increasing percentage of subjects that is overweight (fig. 1): at age 13 less than 1% is overweight but at 36 years 43% of the males and 25% of the females have a BMI >25. These BMI values are comparable with recent data from the MORGEN study [22] in which in a random sample of the Dutch population the prevalence of risk indicators is monitored. The population from the AGAHLS can therefore be considered as representative for the Dutch population. Also other characteristics such as social-economic status showed levels that are only slightly higher than the average Dutch population [9]. Although the prevalence

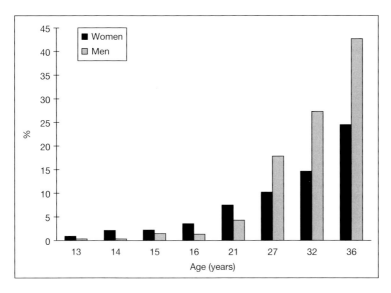

Fig. 1. The percentage of males and females with a body mass index (BMI) above 25 kg/m^2 from age 13 till 36 years.

of obesity is high, one must take into account that the majority of the males and females do show values of their fat mass that are in the normal range and are not showing any degree of obesity or overweight according the criteria of the World Health Organization [1].

BMI and S4S show relatively good tracking, with coefficients of 0.70–0.75, that are equal to that of serum cholesterol (0.71), but higher than those of other CVD risk indicators as systolic and diastolic blood pressure (0.43 and 0.34) [19]. The high tracking of fat mass is an important finding because this knowledge indicates the relevance to aim intervention towards this biological parameter early in adolescence. The low tracking of DI and PA [19] demonstrates that these lifestyle parameters are less stable. Part of the low stability may be caused by the lack of reliability of the measurement method of these lifestyles by interview. Low tracking suggests that interventions should be given to the public as a whole, and not only to those with unhealthy PA or DI values.

In 2000, total body fat was measured for the first time at age 36 years with Dual X-Ray Absorptiometry (DEXA). Post hoc, these data were now used in order to check if the found PA and DI relationships with S4S, measuring only fat from skinfolds, is different from the PA and DI relationships with total body fat percentage (Fat%). The results of these cross-sectional analyses that are comparable to the longitudinal analyses regarding the actual values of table 2 are presented in table 3. It is shown that the regression coefficients of DI and

Table 3. Regression coefficients (mean and 95% CI) of dietary intake (DI, z-scores) and physical activity (PA, z-scores) with sum of four skinfolds (S4S, cm), body mass index (BMI, kg/m²), and body fat percentage (Fat%, measured with DEXA) of men and women measured at age 36 years

			b	95% CI	p value
PA	Men	S4S	−0.14	−0.37; 0.09	0.24
		BMI	−0.20	−0.62; 0.21	0.34
		Fat%	−0.73	−1.68; 0.22	0.13
	Women	S4S	0.30	0.03; 0.57	0.03
		BMI	0.58	0.12; 1.04	0.01
		Fat%	1.02	0.04; 2.00	0.04
DI	Men	S4S	−0.25	−0.48; −0.01	0.04
		BMI	−0.11	−0.53; 0.31	0.61
		Fat%	−1.62	−2.57; −0.68	0.001
	Women	S4S	−0.29	−0.56; −0.02	0.04
		BMI	−0.33	−0.79; 0.13	0.16
		Fat%	−1.57	−2.54; 0.60	0.002

PA with S4S (and BMI) are similar to those with Fat%. The regression coefficients of PA and DI have the same direction for Fat% as for S4S and BMI: expected negative relationships in men with PA, and unexpected positive relationships in women with PA. With DI all relationships are negative and unexpected. Alike for DI, the unexpected positive relationship in women, between PA and body composition at age 36 years may be caused by differential misreport (i.e., through PA over-report of those with high a fat%).

The literature on the relation of both lifestyles PA and DI with body composition is scarce in this age group and gives a variety of results: cross sectional studies resulted in inverse relations [23–26]. One intervention study [27] showed no relation and a case-control study resulted in an inverse relation [28]. The reviews by Parizkova et al. [29] and Roberts et al. [30] and the meta-analysis of Ballor et al. [31] in general conclude that obesity in adolescents only can be altered by increasing PA and decreasing DI.

From the present results it can be concluded that PA levels and changes are negatively related with the levels and changes in the S4S and BMI in males but not females, over the age period from 13 through 36 years. A low or a decrease in DI however is not related to a low or a decrease in BMI and S4S. Therefore, the promotion of physical activity may be more effective than the promotion of low DI, in bringing the energy intake and energy output in balance to achieve the necessary early prevention of obesity.

References

1 Seidell JC, Rissanen AM: Time trends in the worldwide prevalence of obesity; in Bray GA, Bouchard C, James WPT (eds): Handbook of Obesity. New York, Marcel Dekker, 1998, pp 79–91.
2 Volksgezondheid Toekomst Verkenning: De som der delen (in Dutch). Rijksinstituut voor Volksgezondheid en Milieu. Utrecht, Elsevier/Tijdstroom, 1997.
3 Gortmaker SL, Dietz WH, Sobol AM, Wehler CA: Increasing pediatric obesity in the United States. Am J Dis Child 1987;141:535–540.
4 Després J-P, Moorjani S, Lupien PJ, Tremblay A, Nadeau A, Bouchard C: Regional distribution of body fat, plasma lipoproteins, and cardiovascular disease. Arteriosclerosis 1990;10:497–511.
5 Kolata G: Obese children: A growing problem. Science 1986;232:20–21.
6 Guo SS, Roche AF, Chumlea WC, Gardner JD, Siervogel RM: The predictive value of childhood body mass index values for overweight at age 35. Am J Clin Nutr 1994;59:810–819.
7 Parsons TJ, Power C, Logan S, Summerbell CD: Childhood predictors of adult obesity: A systematic review. Int J Obes 1999;23(suppl 8):S1–S107.
8 Bray GA, Bouchard C, James WPT: Handbook of Obesity. New York, Marcel Dekker, 1998.
9 Kemper HCG (ed): Growth health and fitness of teenagers: Longitudinal research in international perspective. Med Sport Sci. Basel, Karger, 1985, vol 20.
10 Kemper HCG (ed): The Amsterdam Growth Study, a longitudinal analysis of health, fitness, and lifestyle. HK Sport Science Monograph. Champaign, Human Kinetics, 1995, vol 6.
11 Weiner JS, Lourie JA: Human Biology: A Guide to Field Methods. IBP Handbook No 9. Oxford, Blackwell, 1969, pp 8–29.
12 Durnin JVGA, Rahaman MM: The assessment of the amount of fat in human body measurements of skinfold thickness. Br J Nutr 1967;21:681–689.
13 Post GB: Nutrition in adolescence: A longitudinal study in dietary patterns from teenager to adult; PhD thesis, Agricultural University of Wageningen, De Vrieseborch, Haarlem, 1989, SO 16.
14 Dutch Food and Nutrition Table (in Dutch): Zeist, Stichting, NEVO, Voorlichtingsburo voor de Voeding, 1985.
15 Verschuur R: Daily physical activity and health: Longitudinal changes during the teenage period; PhD thesis, University of Amsterdam, De Vrieseborch, Haarlem, 1987, SO 12.
16 Montoye HJ, Kemper HCG, Saris WHM, Washburn RA: Measuring Physical Activity and Energy Expenditure. Champaign, Human Kinetics, 1996, pp 123–183.
17 Bakker I, Twisk JWR, van Mechelen W, Mensink GBM, Kemper HCG: Computerization of a dietary history interview in a running cohort; evaluation within the Amsterdam Growth and Health Longitudinal Study. Eur J Clin Nutr 2003;57:394–404.
18 Twisk JWR, Kemper HCG, van Mechelen W, Post GB: Which lifestyle parameters discriminate high- from low-risk participants for coronary heart disease risk factors: Longitudinal analysis covering adolescence and young adulthood. J Cardiovasc Risk 1997;4:393–400.
19 Twisk JWR, Kemper HCG, van Mechelen W, Post GB: Tracking of risk factors for coronary disease over a 14-period: A comparison between lifestyle and biologic risk factors with data from the Amsterdam Growth and Health Study. Am J Epidemiol 1997;145,10:889–898.
20 Goris AH, Westerterp-Plantinga MS, Westerterp KR: Undereating and underrecording of habitual food intake in obese men: selective underreporting of fat intake. Am J Clin Nutr 2000;71,1:130–134.
21 Kemper HCG, van Mechelen W, Post GB, Snel J, Twisk JWR, van Lenthe FJ, Welten DC: The Amsterdam Growth and Health Longitudinal Study, the past (1976–1996) and future (1997–?). Int J Sports Med 1997;18:S141–S150.
22 Blokstra A, Seidell JC, Smit AH, Bueno de Mesquita HB, Verschuren WMM: Morgen Project (in Dutch). Bilthoven, RIVM, 1997.
23 Fripp RR, Hodgson JL, Kwiterovich PO, Werner JC, Schuler HG, Whitman V: Aerobic capacity, obesity and artherosclerotic risk factors in male adolescents. Pediatrics 1985;75:813.
24 Pena M, Baccallao J, Barta L, Amador M, Johnston FE: Fiber and exercise in the treatment of obese adolescents. J Adolesc Health Care 1989;10:30–34.
25 Bandini LG, Schoeller DA, Dietz WH: Energy expenditure in obese and non obese adolescents. Pediatr Res 1990;27:198–203.

26   Roberts SB, Young VR, Fuss P, Heyman MB, Fiatarone M, Dallal GE, Evans WJ: What are the dietary energy needs of elderly adults? Int J Obes 1992;16:969–976.
27   Blaak EE, Westerterp KR, Bar-Or O, Wouters LJM, Saris WHM: Total energy expenditure and spontaneous activity in relation to training in obese boys. Am J Clin Nutr 1992;55:777–782.
28   Moussa MAA, Skaik MB, Yaghy OY: Factors associated with obesity in school children. Int J Obes 1994;18:513–515.
29   Parizkova J: Physical training in weight reduction of obese adolescents. Am J Clin Res 1982;34: 63–68.
30   Roberts SB: Abnormalities of energy expenditure and the development of obesity. Obes Res 1995;3.
31   Ballor DL, Keessey RE: A meta-analysis of the factors affecting exercise-induced changes in body mass, fat mass and fat-free mass in males and females. Int J Obes 1991;15:717–726.

Prof. Dr. Han C.G. Kemper
AGAHLS Research Group, EMGO Institute
VU University Medical Center
Van der Boechorststraat 7, NL–1081 BT Amsterdam (The Netherlands)
Tel. +31 20 4448407, Fax +31 20 4446775, E-Mail hcg.kemper.emgo@med.vu.nl

Kemper HCG (ed): Amsterdam Growth and Health Longitudinal Study.
Med Sport Sci. Basel, Karger, 2004, vol 47, pp 153–166

....

Is Physical Activity Important for Aerobic Power in Young Males and Females?

Han C.G. Kemper, Lando L.J. Koppes

Institute for Research in Extramural Medicine (EMGO Institute),
VU University Medical Center, Amsterdam, The Netherlands

Abstract

Background/Aims: The purpose of this paper is to test the hypothesis that physical activity (PA), measured over a period of 23 years is beneficial to aerobic power (VO_2max) in young males and females (13–36 years) from the Amsterdam Growth and Health Longitudinal Study (AGAHLS). ***Methods:*** PA was measured using heart rate and pedometer monitoring and a standardized activity interview. VO_2max was assessed with a maximal running test on a treadmill. To assess the longitudinal relationship between PA and VO_2max five different longitudinal analyses are carried out over different age periods, correcting for various confounders such as lifestyle parameters, biological parameters, and initial VO_2max. ***Results:*** Highly significant relationships were observed between PA and VO_2max in four of the five analyses. However, when present PA is related to the future change in VO_2max, the results are not significant. ***Conclusion:*** Data from the AGAHLS population does not fully support the hypothesis that PA effects VO_2max.

Hypoactivity is believed to be a direct and indirect cause of many pediatric diseases [1] but also for adult chronic diseases such as cardiovascular diseases (CVD), type 2 diabetes, osteoporosis, and several types of cancer [2]. The high prevalence of hypoactivity is striking. Caspersen [3], for example, estimated that 59% of the United States population fails to perform regular leisuretime physical activity. This prevalence is much higher than for the three traditional CVD risk factors. For hypercholesterolemia the prevalence is 19%, for cigarette smoking 18%, and for high blood pressure only 10%. The increase in relative risk (RR) for each of the four CVD risk factors is of similar magnitude: The RR varies from 1.9 (physical inactivity) to 2.5 (cigarette smoking). Mostly due to the high prevalence, the population attributable risk (PAR) for physical inactivity on all-cause mortality and CVD mortality is the highest [4]. Therefore, physical activity appears to be a more important concern for its population impact than the other three mentioned risk factors [3]. The importance of PA in the prevention of CVD mortality lately is entering reports that are close to policy makers. In the Netherlands, physical inactivity is recognized as an important lifestyle factor in the contribution to CVD mortality [5].

Next to the association between physical activity and CVD an even stronger association has been demonstrated between aerobic power and CVD, with the risk for CVD mortality of the least fit generally being at least fivefold as high as the risk for the most fit [6–10]. The study of Lakka et al. [11] concluded that aerobic power was protective against CVD only in physically active individuals. The majority of the studies show that the greatest differences in CVD rates are found between the least active or fit and the moderately active or fit individuals, with little additional benefit seen with additional activity or fitness, suggesting a threshold effect. This is also in agreement with the data from the Multiple Risk Factor Intervention Trial (MRFIT), as described by Leon et al. [12]. However, a meta-analysis by Berlin and Golditz [13] demonstrated a more stable dose-response relationship between the intensity of the physical activity and CVD risks: a lower relative risk for CVD risk indicators and lower CVD mortality rate was related with a higher intensity of physical activity in the included studies.

It is often suggested that a sufficient amount and intensity of regular physical activity during youth could decelerate the development of low fitness, disease and mortality [12]. However, a prospective study comparing physically active children with less active children over a long period of time in a randomized controlled trial (RCT) cannot be executed due to ethical constraints. In an effort to overcome this problem, in this chapter we tested the plausibility of the causality of the relationship using observational longitudinal data from a group of males and females who were monitored over a period of 23 years on their pattern of physical activity and aerobic power. To get an indication of a possible effect of this long-term pattern of physical activity on aerobic power, longitudinal analyses are carried out over different age periods (13–16, 13–27 and 13–36 years). Since aerobic power of the subjects at the start of the study could bias the effect of physical activity, the analyses were corrected for initial aerobic fitness at age 13 years, enabling to draw quasi-causal conclusions.

Methods

The Amsterdam Growth and Health Longitudinal Study (AGAHLS) used a multiple longitudinal design [14]. In this design repeated measurements were done in three birth cohorts (1962, 1963 and 1964) of males and females from a secondary school in Amsterdam [15]. Between 1976 and 2000, nine repeated measurements of PA, fitness and many other variables were completed. Four annual measurements during the school period (at mean ages of 13, 14, 15 and 16 respectively), a fifth in 1985 (at a mean age of 21 years) a sixth measurement in 1991 (mean age 27 years) and a seventh in 1993 (age 29 years) [16]. In 1996 (age 32) and in 2000 (age 36), the last two measurements took place.

In view of the many confounding effects inevitably connected to longitudinal measurements, cohort effects, time of measurement effects and testing effects were estimated for all the measured variables separately [17, 18]. The two parameters of interest in this paper (aerobic power and physical activity) did not show statistically significant repeated testing effects, differences between cohorts, or time-points of measurements in both males and females [19]. Also the drop outs (24% after the first four measurements and 9% after the fifth measurement) were not different from those that remained in the study. For example their body mass index (BMI), as an indication of aerobic fitness and physical activity level showed no significantly higher levels in comparison with the longitudinal group [16].

Physical Activity (PA)

During the adolescent period, PA was monitored by heart rate and pedometer during week-end days [20]. The method applied over the complete 23-year longitudinal period was a standardized activity interview based on a questionnaire [21]. The interview was the same over the years and took place each time in the same period of the year (between February and June) and was retrospective over the previous 3 months. The physical activities that came under review covered the following areas: organized sports activities, unorganized sports activities, active transportation to and from school, work, etc., and work and home activities [22]. Only those activities were taken into account, which had duration of at least 5 min and an intensity level of more than four times the basal metabolic rate (MET). Activities below 4 METs were not reported because they contribute very little to aerobic power [23]. The physical activities were classified as light (4–7 METs), medium-heavy (7–10 METs), and heavy (>10 METs) based on the literature [24]. For the purpose of scoring, the METs assigned to these categories were 5.5, 8.5 and 11.5, respectively. The interview assessed the average weekly time spent doing activities in each of the three categories. MET scores per week were derived through a multiplication of the average time spent per week (min) in each category with the respective MET value for that category. The scores of the three levels were added to arrive to a score of total METs times minutes per week: Weighted Activity Score $= (5.5 \cdot \text{min/week}) + (8.5 \cdot \text{min/week}) + (11.5 \cdot \text{min/week})$, in METs/week. This weighted activity score is used as a combined measure of the duration and intensity of the daily physical activity of the subjects for each year of measurement [21]. In the year 2000, the interview was computerized and as a consequence this influenced the mean results. In order to be able to use the data in a longitudinal manner, z-scores were calculated.

Aerobic Power (VO_2max)

VO_2max was measured by a running test on a treadmill (Quinton, model 18-54). A standard protocol was used with a submaximal test preceding a maximal test. The submaximal test consisted of three 2-min runs at a constant speed of 8 km/h, with slopes of 0, 2.5 and 5% (in that order). During practice for this 6 min submaximal running, the subjects warmed up, got accustomed to running on the treadmill, and were acquainted with the mouthpiece and noseclip, needed for the measurement of oxygen uptake. After a short period of rest

(10–15 min), running was continued on the same treadmill at the same constant speed of 8 km/h. In this maximal test the slope was increased every 2 min by 2.5 or 5% depending on the heart rate (HR) of the subject. The Ergoanalyzer (Jaeger, Bunnik, The Netherlands) continuously and automatically analyzed the collected expired air and calculated minute ventilation (VE), and oxygen uptake (VO_2), standardized for temperature, humidity and barometric pressure (STPD). Measurement of the VO_2 with the Ergoanalyzer was used at each time point. This assessment method has proven to be comparable to the classical method of collecting expired air in Douglas bags and analyzing carbon dioxide and oxygen content with the Scholander technique [25]. The maximal running test was continued until complete exhaustion had been reached. Each subject was encouraged verbally to exercise to his or her maximum.

The maximal oxygen uptake (VO_2max) was taken as criterion for aerobic power. VO_2max (ml · min^{-1}) is the highest mean minute value of the VO_2 during the maximal running test. VO_2max is a complicated variable. First of all this is the case because of the need for a reliable metabolic analysis system of the respiration during running. Secondly, because VO_2max during growth depends on body size, and VO_2max expressed per kilogram of body weight is still strongly related to body weight [26]. Therefore, we also expressed VO_2max according the allometric scaling approach [27], being relative to body weight to the two-thirds power (ml · min^{-1} · kg body weight$^{-2/3}$). The effectiveness of this treadmill test in reaching a true maximal oxygen uptake was evaluated from the maximal heart rate (more than 95% of the predicted maximum corrected for age) and the respiratory gas exchange ratio (a value of more than 1.0). The classic definition of a VO_2 plateau was not used, because it is proven that at least in children and adolescents those who plateau do not have higher VO_2, heart rate or blood lactate value than those not demonstrating a VO_2 plateau [28].

Different Periods, Different Analyses

In this chapter, different analyses are used to evaluate the question: Is physical activity important for aerobic power?

First, we regrouped the boys and girls into active and inactive groups based on the four annual measurements in their teenage period (13–16 years). The selection was based on three PA variables: (a) energy expenditure measured from heart rate recording over 48 h [29]; (b) pedometer week-scores [30], and (c) total time spent per week (above 4 MET) according the standardized activity interview [21]. The active boys and girls were those who scored above the median (P50) in at least two of the three activity measurements per year, and in at least three out of four annual measurements [31].

Second, we analyzed with multiple analysis of variance (MANOVA) the longitudinal relationship between PA and VO_2max over a period of 14 years (from age 13 till age 27), using activity data that are based on the interview. VO_2max values of the relatively high active subjects of each sex (those in the top tertile) were compared with those of the relatively inactive subjects (those in the bottom tertile).

Third, over the same period, standardized regression coefficients were calculated using generalized estimating equations (GEE). With GEE [32], the longitudinal relationships were analyzed using all available PA and VO_2max data and under correction of both time-dependent (biological age, biologic and lifestyle variables) and time-independent (gender) covariates. Furthermore, the method takes into account that the repeated observations of an individual are not independent. In the AGAHLS this method has been used successfully to analyze the longitudinal relationships between biological and lifestyle coronary heart disease

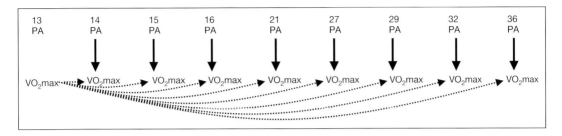

Fig. 1. Representation of the regression model of physical activity (PA) on aerobic power (VO$_2$max) with correction for initial VO$_2$max.

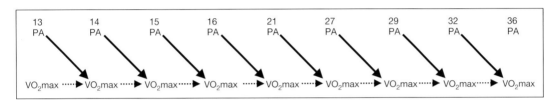

Fig. 2. Representation of the auto-regression model of present physical activity (PA) on future VO$_2$max with correction for present VO$_2$max.

risk factors [33, 34]. GEE with a continuous outcome variable (VO$_2$max) is comparable to a (longitudinal) linear regression analysis. As a result, standardized regression coefficients can be calculated.

Fourth, it can be assumed that the longitudinal relation between physical activity on the one hand and aerobic power on the other hand also depends on the initial aerobic power of the subject. Subjects with a relatively high aerobic fitness at the age of 13 years should increase their VO$_2$max less than subjects with a relatively low initial aerobic fitness. Therefore, in these statistical analysis we corrected for initial VO$_2$max measured on the first measurement, when the males and females were 13 years old (fig. 1).

Fifth, we analyzed with GEE all available PA and VO$_2$max data over the total period of 23 years from age 13 till age 36, in an autoregressive model. Herein we calculated the longitudinal relation of present PA on the VO$_2$max value of the next measurement, with correction for the present VO$_2$max value (fig. 2). These analyses give an answer to the question whether or not a difference in activity level results in a change in VO$_2$max.

For all analyses, a 5% significance level was used. The GEE analysis were carried out with the Statistical Package for Interactive Data Analysis (SPIDA) [35] and the other (MANOVA and linear regression analyses) with the Statistical Package for the Social Sciences [36].

Covariates Used in the Statistical Analyses

With a crosscheck dietary interview [37, 38] the individual daily food intake of the subjects was estimated. Based on the Dutch Food and Nutrition table [39] total energy intake, the relative energetic contributions of fat, carbohydrate and protein were calculated. Systolic and diastolic blood pressure was measured with a sphygmomanometer in the arteria brachialis with the participants at rest in the sitting position. For the determination of total cholesterol in serum, 10 ml of venous blood, taken from the vena antecubitus was analyzed and validated with control samples from a World Health Organization reference laboratory. Body fat mass was estimated as the sum of four skinfolds at the biceps, triceps, subscapular and suprailiac locations with a Harpenden skinfold caliper [40]. During the first 4 years as a measure of biological maturation, skeletal age was estimated from the X-ray of the left hand [41]. After full maturation (girls at age 16 and boys at age 18), at ages 21, 27, 29, 32 and 36 years, calendar age was used as indicator for biological maturation.

Results

In table 1, the means and standard deviations of anthropometrics (body height, body weight), daily physical activity, maximal aerobic power (VO_2max) are summarized for males and females at age 13, 16, 21, 27, 32 and 36. The mean growth over the 23-year period in height of males is about 24 cm and in females about 9 cm. The adult height and weight of the males and females at age 36 do not differ from the standard Dutch population [42]. PA decreased significantly from 4,700 METs/week in boys and 3,800 METs/week in girls at age 13 to about 3,000 METs/week in both men and women at age 27. At age 32, there was a small trend in both sexes of an increase to 3,400 METs/week and at age 36 the level of PA has further increased. When considered allometrically, VO_2max decreased gradually in females from 185 to 160 ml $\cdot$ min^{-1} $\cdot$ kg$^{-2/3}$. In males it increased during the teenage period from 210 to 233 and a trend of a decrease thereafter to 212 ml $\cdot$ min^{-1} $\cdot$ kg$^{-2/3}$ was seen at age 27. At age 36, both sexes again showed increased VO_2max values.

The Adolescent Period (13–16 Years)
In figure 3, the mean values of VO_2max relative to body weight are shown of boys and girls divided in active and inactive ones. The active boys and girls show higher VO_2max values than the inactive ones, but the differences are small and the inactive adolescents still have a reasonable VO_2max during the whole adolescent period (males 56 ml/kg/min, females 45 ml/kg/min).

The 14-Year Period (13–27 Years)
By MANOVA for repeated measures the relatively high active subjects (>P67) are compared with the relatively low active subjects (<P33) on their VO_2max relative to their body mass to the 2/3 power (VO_2max/BM$^{2/3}$). In both sexes, the relatively high physically active groups showed significantly higher

Table 1. Means and standard deviations of body height, body weight, daily physical activity and maximal aerobic power (VO_2max) in males and females at ages 13, 16, 21 and 27

	Height cm		Weight kg		Physical activity kMETs		VO_2max ml/kg/min	
	♂	♀	♂	♀	♂	♀	♂	♀
13 n	314	337	316	340	195	214	195	215
Mean	160	161	43.2	46.5	4.7	3.8	59.1	51.2
(SD)	(83)	(75)	(7.5)	(8.3)	(2.0)	(1.7)	(6.0)	(6.2)
16 n	217	278	222	280	140	173	139	165
Mean	179	169	60.9	57.1	3.7	3.2	58.4	45.6
(SD)	(71)	(63)	(8.4)	(7.6)	(1.9)	(1.5)	(5.8)	(4.7)
21 n	93	107	93	107	93	107	93	105
Mean	183	170	71.4	62.4	3.6	3.3	53.5	41.1
(SD)	(62)	(65)	(8.3)	(9.3)	(2.5)	(2.1)	(5.5)	(4.2)
27 n	84	98	84	98	84	98	84	93
Mean	183	170	75.5	63.3	2.9	3.2	50.5	40.5
(SD)	(66)	(61)	(8.4)	(7.8)	(2.3)	(1.9)	(5.7)	(5.0)
32 n	205	232	205	232	206	232	201	228
Mean	184	170	81.0	65.4	3.3	3.5	46.1	40.1
(SD)	(62)	(65)	(9.9)	(9.1)	(2.3)	(2.4)	(6.9)	(6.1)
36 n	178	200	178	200	178	199	174	190
Mean	184	170	83.8	67.9	4.4	5.4	51.1	40.8
(SD)	(65)	(63)	(10.7)	(10.2)	(2.7)	(3.7)	(7.4)	(6.1)

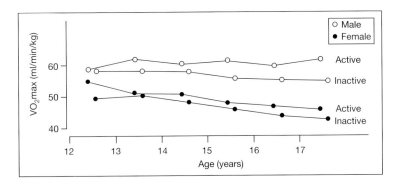

Fig. 3. Development of VO_2max per body mass (VO_2max/BM) in boys and girls with relatively high (active) and low (inactive) patterns during the adolescent period.

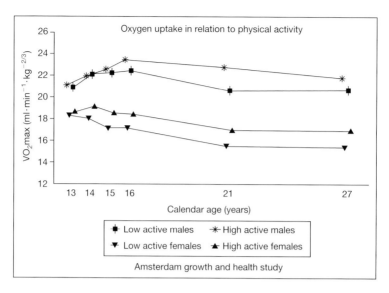

Fig. 4. Comparison of relatively high active males and females (>P67) with their low active peers (<P33) with respect to maximal oxygen uptake (VO₂max) between 13 and 27 years of age.

VO₂max (fig. 4). This indicates that over these 14 years of follow-up, the highly active males and females developed a higher VO₂max compared to their less active counterparts.

The results of the longitudinal GEE analyses are presented in table 2. In the crude analysis a highly significant longitudinal relationship between weighted physical activity score on the one hand and aerobic power (VO₂max) on the other was found. This univariate analysis was corrected for gender, time of measurement and the initial value of VO₂max at age 13 years. The magnitude of the relationships was significant, but relatively small (beta = 0.09), indicating that a 30% higher activity level is related with a 0.09 2% higher VO₂max. Correcting for lifestyle parameters (adjusted 1) or for biological parameters (adjusted 2) did not have much influence on the strength of the relationship. No significant interaction effects with biological age and gender could be demonstrated. Further analyses about possible interactions of smoking and fatness did not result in any significant findings.

The Total Period of 23 Years (13–36 Years)

The results of the GEE analysis over the 23-year period based on the model outlined in figure 1 was in line with the former results. A highly significant, but small, relationship was found. A 10% difference in MET score was positively

Table 2. Standardized regression coefficients and p values obtained by generalized estimating equations regarding the longitudinal relationship between weighted physical activity on the one hand and VO₂max and maximal slope on the other

Analysis	VO_2max β	p value	Maximal slope β	p value
Crude	0.09	<0.01	0.10	<0.01
Adjusted 1	0.08	<0.01	0.10	<0.01
Adjusted 2	0.07	<0.01	0.08	<0.01

Crude = 'Univariate' analysis (correcting for gender time and initial value of either VO₂max or maximal slope); adjusted 1 = multiple analysis like crude also correcting for lifestyle parameters; adjusted 2 = multiple analysis like crude also correcting for biological parameters.

related to a 0.3% difference in VO₂max (95% confidence interval (CI): 0.2–0.4). In contrast, the analyses based on the autoregressive model outlined in figure 2, in which was controlled for present VO₂max, revealed that a difference in activity level of 10% was positively related a nonsignificant difference in VO₂max of only 0.04% (95% CI: −0.06 to 0.13).

Discussion

The results of the analyses of the longitudinal relationship between daily physical activity and aerobic power over 3-, 14- and 23-year periods in a normal young healthy population, with and without correction for initial aerobic power, or other confounders (such as smoking, alcohol consumption, dietary intake), are highly significant. Although these longitudinal associations are in the expected direction, the changes in VO₂max are relatively small. The longitudinal associations that were found can not be interpreted as a causal relationship, because of the fact that the collected data are observational [17]. Furthermore, the relationship was even absent in the last and most sophisticated analysis over the whole period. In this last analysis, current physical activity level were regressed on future VO₂max, correcting for current fitness (fig. 2). This last model therefore concerns the question if VO₂max follows activity.

Stability of Physical Activity and Aerobic Fitness
One of the possible explanations for these results can be a relatively high intra-individual stability within subjects of daily physical activity and aerobic fitness over the age period under consideration. However, in earlier publications

(and in the chapter by Koppes et al. [pp 44–63]) we have shown that the relative stability of daily physical activity was quite low. Van Mechelen et al. [22] found 15-year interperiod correlation coefficients for daily physical activity of 0.17 for males and 0.05 for females. Twisk et al. [43] used a different approach and calculated over the same time period a 'longitudinal' tracking coefficient for daily physical activity of 0.34 (95% confidence interval 0.19–0.49). The stability of aerobic fitness is of the same magnitude as the relative stability for daily physical activity, with a longitudinal tracking coefficient of 0.31 (95% confidence interval 0.24–0.38) [43]. In other words, there is no relatively high intra-individual stability for both physical activity and aerobic fitness, so this cannot explain the present findings [44].

In an 8-year follow-up study, Andersen et al. [45] measured physical activity (participation in sporting activities during leisure time) and VO_2max in 16- to 19-year-old Danish boys and girls. The 8-year inter-period correlation coefficients of VO_2max were 0.35 in boys and 0.48 in girls, while those and of physical activity were even lower: 0.31 in boys and 0.20 in girls. Their tracking coefficients, covering only half of our longitudinal period, are comparable to the ones in the present study. In the same study, changes over 8 years in physical activity appeared not to be correlated with changes in VO_2max [45].

These results are not in accordance with our findings, but can be explained by the fact that the magnitude of the relationship is relatively small, and that statistical significance was attained in the present study, and not in that of Andersen and Haraldsdottir [45], because of a difference in statistical power. We had a larger number of participants, and nine repeated measurements between age 13 and 36 years, as compared with only one measurement at the beginning and one at the end in the Danish study.

Physical Activity

Daily physical activity is a complex phenomenon, because intensity, duration, and frequency characterize it [21]. In this longitudinal study it was measured using a cross-check interview taking into account intensity, duration and frequency of daily activities. This way of measuring the amount and intensity of daily physical activity can, at its best, only be a rough estimate of the real daily physical activity [46].

The standardized interview was assessed nine times with almost the same protocol over the 23 years. In the first 4 years we compared the activity interview data with data from the same subjects of 48-hour heart rate and pedometer registrations [15]. Pearson correlation coefficients between the MET score from the physical activity interviews on the one hand and the heart rate recording and the pedometer score on the other hand were significant, but small, in both sexes [13]. However, with values between 16 and 20, they explain little of one another's variation. The interview appears to give a more global estimate, but is influenced by the memory of the subject. The heart rate and pedometer measurements are more valid in this respect but are only monitored over 2–4 days. Moreover, pedometers attached to the waist do not register activities such as bicycling and heart rate can also be elevated by other sources than activity such as stress and heat. Therefore, we believe that in the present study daily physical activity was assessed in the most accurate way available at this time.

Implications of the Results

It should be noted that the huge decrease in physical activity levels from adolescence into young adulthood could have important public health implications regarding the risk for CVD. In the same population it was found that a relatively high physical activity was highly associated with favorable HDL-levels in blood and to low body fatness [33]. So the drop in physical activity levels can be associated to an unfavorable CVD risk profile at adult age.

The standardized regression coefficients regarding the longitudinal relationship between PA and VO_2max over the 15-year period (table 2) can also be functionally transformed. An increase of 1,000 METs/week is related to an increase of $4 \, ml \cdot min^{-1} \cdot kg^{-2/3}$ in VO_2max. Although the strength of the observed relationship between physical activity and aerobic fitness was highly significant, the functional implications seem less impressive: an increase of 30% in PA (equals approximately 1,000 METs/week) during a period of 15 years, resulted in an increase of only 2% in VO_2max. Moreover, if we take into account that the relationship calculated with autoregression over the period of 23 years resulted in nonsignificant relationships, we must admit that in this observational study no clear relation can be proved between PA and VO_2max in free living males and females.

Conclusion

From this study it can be concluded that during adolescence and (young) adulthood daily PA is strongly related to VO_2max. The direction of the observed relationship remains unclear and possible functional implications are small, because in the 23-year longitudinal analysis, taking into consideration present PA on future VO_2max with correction for present VO_2max, the expected positive relationship was not significant. This may indicate that genetic factors [47] are more important than environmental factors in the question about the importance of physical activity for aerobic power, or that the effect of PA on VO_2max is that short-lived that it is not detectable with the longitudinal AGAHLS data that were gathered with time intervals of at least 1 year.

References

1   Bar-Or O: Pediatric Sports Medicine, from Physiologic Principles to Clinical Applications. New York, Springer, 1984, pp 66–73.
2   US Department of Health and Human Services: The effects of physical activity on health and disease; in: Physical Activity and Health. A Report of the Surgeon General. Pittsburgh, Superintendent of Documents, 1996, pp 81–172.
3   Caspersen CJ: Physical activity epidemiology concepts, methods and applications to exercise science. Exerc Sport Sci Rev 1989;17:423–473.
4   Powell KE, Thompson PD, Caspersen CJ, Kendrick JS: Physical activity and the incidence of coronary heart diseases. Ann Rev Publ Hlth 1987;8:253–287.
5   Ruwaard D, Kramers PGN (eds): Volksgezondheid, Toekomst Verkenning 1997. De som der delen, Rijks Instituut voor Volksgezondheid en Milieu, Utrecht. Amsterdam, Elsevier/De Tijdstroom, 1997.
6   Bijnen FCH, Caspersen CL, Mosterd WL: Physical inactivity as a risk factor for coronary heart disease: A WHO and International Society and Federation of Cardiology position statement. Bull Wld Hlth Org 1994;72,1:1–4.
7   Blair SN, Kampert JB, Kohl HW, Barlow CE, Macera CA, Paffenbarger RS, Gibbons LW: Influences of cardiorespiratory fitness and other precursors on cardiorespiratory disease and all-cause mortality in men and women. JAMA 1996;276:205–210.
8   Blair SN, Kohl HW, Paffenbarger RS, Clark DG, Cooper KH, Gillbons LW: Physical fitness and all-cause mortality: A prospective study on healthy men and women. JAMA 1989;262:2395–2401.
9   Lee IM, Paffenbarger RS: Do physical activity and physical fitness avert premature mortality?; in Holloszy JJ (ed): Exercise and Sport Sciences Reviews. Baltimore, Williams & Wilkins, 1996, vol 24, pp 135–171.
10 Paffenbarger RS Jr, Hyde RT, Wing AL, Hsieh V: Physical activity, all cause mortality and longevity of college alumni. N Engl J Med 1986;314:606–613.
11 Lakka TA, Veralinen JM, Rauramaa R, Salonen R, Tuomlehto J, Salonen JT: Relation of leisure-time physical activity and cardiorespiratory fitness to risk of acute myocardial infarction. N Engl J Med 1994;330:1549–1554.
12 Leon AS, Meyers MJ, Connett J: Leisure time physical activity and the 16-year risks of mortality from coronary heart disease and all-causes in the multiple risk factor intervention trial (MRFIT). Int J Sports Med 1997;18:s208–s215.
13 Berlin JA, Colditz GA: A meta-analysis of physical activity in the prevention of coronary heart disease. Am J Epidemiol 1990;132:612–628.
14 Kemper HCG, van 't Hof MA: Design of a multiple longitudinal interdisciplinary study of growth and health in teenagers. Eur J Pediatr 1978;129:147–155.
15 Kemper HCG (ed): Growth, health and fitness of teenagers, longitudinal research in international perspective. Med Sport Sci. Basel, Karger, 1985, vol 20.
16 Kemper HCG (ed): The Amsterdam Growth Study: A Longitudinal Analysis of Health, Fitness, and Lifestyle. HK Sport Science Monograph Series. Champaign, Human Kinetics, 1995, vol 6.
17 Kemper HCG: The Amsterdam Growth and Health Longitudinal Study: The past (1976–1996) and future (1997–?). Int J Sports Med 1997;18:s140–s150.
18 Kemper HCG: The natural history of physical activity and aerobic fitness in teenagers; in Dishman RK (ed): Advances in Exercise Adherence. Champaign, Human Kinetics, 1994, vol 11, pp 293–318.
19 Kemper HCG: Sources of variation in longitudinal assessment of maximal aerobic power in teenage boys and girls: The Amsterdam Growth and Health Study. Hum Biol 1991;63,4: 533–546.

20   Kemper HCG, Bom C vd, Dekker H, Ootjers G, Post B, Snel J, Splinter PG, Storm-van Essen L, Verschuur R: Growth and health of Teenagers in The Netherlands. Survey of multidisciplinary longitudinal studies and comparison with recent results of a Dutch study. Int J Sports Med 1983;4: 202–214.

21   Montoye HJ, Kemper HCG, Saris WHM, Washburn RA: Measuring Physical Activity and Energy Expenditure. Champaign, Human Kinetics, 1996, appendix-P, pp 183–184.

22   van Mechelen W, Kemper HCG: Habitual physical activity in longitudinal perspective; in Kemper HCG (ed): The Amsterdam Growth Study, HK Sport Science Monograph Series. Champaign, Human Kinetics, 1995, vol 6, pp 135–158.

23   American College of Sports Medicine: Position statement on the recommended quantity and quality of exercise for developing and maintaining cardiorespiratory and muscular fitness in healthy adults. Med Sci Sports Exerc 1990;22:265–274.

24   Verschuur R: Daily physical activity and health: Longitudinal changes during the teenage period; thesis, University of Amsterdam, De Vrieseborch Haarlem, 1987.

25   Kemper HCG, Binkhorst RA, Verschuur R, Visser ACA: Reliability of the Ergoanalyzer. J Cardiovasc Techn 1976;4:27–30.

26   Åstrand PO, Rodahl K: Textbook of Work Physiology. New York, McGraw Hill, 1986, vol 11, pp 367–388.

27   Welsman J, Armstrong N, Kirby BJ, Neville AM, Winter E: Scaling peak oxygen uptake for differences in body size. Med Sci Sports Exerc 1996;28:259–265.

28   Armstrong N, Welsman JR: Aerobic fitness; in Armstrong N, van Mechelen W (eds): Paediatric Exercise Science and Medicine. Oxford, Oxford University Press, 2000, vol 1.7, pp 65–75.

29   Saris WH, Snel P, Binkhorst RA: A portable heart rate distribution recorder for studying daily physical activity. Eur J Appl Phys Occ Phys 1977;37:19–25.

30   Verschuur R, Kemper HCG: Adjustment of pedometers to make them more valid in assessing running. Int J Sports Med 1980;1:87–89.

31   Kemper HCG: Longitudinal studies on the development of health and fitness and the interaction with physical activity of teenagers. Pediatrician 1986;13:52–59.

32   Zeger SL, Liang K-Y: Longitudinal data analysis for discrete and continuous outcomes. Biometrics 1986;42:121–130.

33   Twisk JWR, Kemper HCG, Mellenbergh GJ, van Mechelen W: Relation between the longitudinal development of lipoprotein levels and biological parameters during adolescence and young adulthood in Amsterdam. J Epidemiol Community Hlth 1996;50:505–511.

34   Twisk JWR, Mellenbergh GJ, van Mechelen W, Post GB: Relation between the longitudinal development of lipoprotein levels and lifestyle parameters during adolescence and young adulthood. Ann Epidemiol 1996;6:246–56.

35   Gebski V, Leung O, McNeil D, Lunn D: Spida User, manual, version 6, Macquarie Univ. N.S.W. Australia, 1992.

36   SPSS-X User's Guide, ed 3. Chicago, SPPS, 1988.

37   Post GB: Nutrition in adolescence: A longitudinal study in dietary patterns from teenage to adult; thesis, Agriculture University Wageningen, De Vrieseborch, Haarlem SO16, 1989.

38   Bakker I, Twisk JWR, van Mechelen W, Mensink GBM, Kemper HCG: Computerization of a dietary history interview in a running cohort: Evaluation within the Amsterdam growth and health longitudinal study. Eur J Clin Nutr 2003;57:394–404.

39   NEVO: Dutch Food Composition Table. The Hague, Stichting NEVO, Voorlichtingsburo van de voeding, 1989.

40   Weiner JS, Lourie JA: Human Biology: A Guide to Field Methods. SBP Handbook Nog. Oxford, Blackwell, 1989.

41   Tanner JM, Whitehouse RH, Marshall WA, Healy MJR, Goldstein H: Assessment of Skeletal Age Maturity and Prediction of Adult Height (TW2 method). London, Academic Press, 1975.

42   Roede MJ, van Wieringen JC: Growth diagrams 1980: Netherlands third nationwide survey. Tijdschr Sociale Gezondheidszorg 1985;63(suppl):1–33.

43   Twisk JWR, Kemper HCG, van Mechelen W, Post GB: Tracking of risk factors for coronary heart disease over a 14-year period: A comparison between lifestyle and biologic risk factors with data from the Amsterdam Growth and Health Study. Am J Epidemiol 1997;145,10:888–898.

44 Twisk JWR, Kemper HCG, van Mechelen W: Tracking of activity and fitness and the relationship with CVD risk factors. Med Sci Sports Exerc 2000;32:1455–1461.

45 Andersen LB, Haraldsdottir J: Changes in physical activity, maximal isometric strength and maximal oxygen uptake from late teenage to adulthood: An eight year follow-up study of adolescents in Denmark. Scand J Med Sci Sports 1994;4:19–25.

46 Montoye HJ: Risk indicators for cardiovascular disease in relation to physical activity in youth; in Binkhorst RA, Kemper HCG, Saris WHM (eds): Children and Exercise: XI International Series on Sport Sciences. Champaign, Human Kinetics, 1985, vol 15, pp 3–26.

47 Bouchard C, Malina RM, Perusse L (eds): Genetics of Fitness and Physical Performance. Champaign, Human Kinetics, 1997.

Prof. Dr. Han C.G. Kemper
AGAHLS Research Group, Institute for Research in Extramural Medicine
VU University Medical Center
Van der Boechorststraat 7, NL–1081 BT Amsterdam (The Netherlands)
Tel. +31 20 4448407, Fax +31 20 4446775, E-Mail hcg.kemper.emgo@med.vu.nl

Kemper HCG (ed): Amsterdam Growth and Health Longitudinal Study.
Med Sport Sci. Basel, Karger, 2004, vol 47, pp 167–182

....

Effects of Health Information in Youth on Adult Biological and Lifestyle Risk Factors for Chronic Diseases

*H.C.G. Kemper[a], L.L.J. Koppes[a], W. de Vente[a], G.B. Post[a],
W. van Mechelen[b], J.W.R. Twisk[a]*

[a] Institute for Research in Extramural Medicine (EMGO Institute), and
[b] Institute for Research in Extramural Medicine and Department of
  Social Medicine, VU University Medical Center, Amsterdam, The Netherlands

Abstract

Background/Aims: In the Amsterdam Growth and Health Longitudinal Study (AGAHLS) data are available to test if lifestyle and biological risk factors for chronic diseases improve due to medical check-ups with personal health information applied over a long period of time. *Methods:* One group of apparently healthy males and females was measured on eight separate occasions between the ages of 13 and 32 years (multi-measured group: MM). At each measurement, participants were given information about their health status. A comparable group was measured at age 13 and 32 only (bi-measured group: BM). *Results:* The 'intervention' appeared to have a positive effect on 2 of the 9 biological risk factors, and 1 of the 20 dietary parameters. Contrary to the hypothesis, a trend for a negative intervention effect was seen on habitual physical activity. *Conclusion:* The limited effects of a 20-year health measurement and information 'intervention' may be due to low contrast between the groups.

More than 65% of total mortality in the population of industrialized countries is due to chronic diseases such as cardiovascular disease (CVD), cancer, diabetes, and chronic obstructive pulmonary disease. The causes of these diseases are multifactorial, having not only genetic [1] but also other biological components (hypertension, hypercholesterolemia, obesity, low physical fitness) [2]. Lifestyle factors, including excess intake of saturated fat, alcohol intake, cigarette smoking, and physical inactivity also contribute substantially to these chronic diseases [3]. The relative risk (RR) of CVD in people with one or more of the risk factors, smoking, obesity, hypercholesterolemia, hypertension and physical inactivity, is 1.9 and 2.5, respectively, as compared with the RR of CVD in people with none of these risk factors [4]. In the Netherlands during the last 20 years the main lifestyle-related CVD risk factors showed a predominantly unfavorable trend and this applied not only to the adult population, but even more so to young people [5].

Theoretical models have been developed to predict changes in health behaviors by linking the determinants of behavior to the actual behavior [6]. In recent years, different psychological theories have been proposed to explain why people engage in health promoting behavior [7]. The readers are referred to Ajzen and Fishbein's [8] theory of planned behavior the Health Belief Model [9], and Prochaska's transtheoretical, or stages of change model [10]. To be successful in the promotion of health and a healthy lifestyle, these models postulate that long-term changes have to be aimed at relevant determinants of health behavior. A number of determinants, such as personality traits and knowledge, only partly explain why people engage in health behaviors. It is also important to consider attitudes, social support, self-efficacy and perceived barriers [8].

Changing lifestyle behaviors in youth is seen as a preventive strategy that can help people to enhance health and avoid chronic diseases during adulthood. Dishman [11] showed that youth may benefit greatly from health promotion programs that focus on physical activity, dietary intake, alcohol consumption, smoking, coping style and subjective health appraisals. Kuh and Cooper [12] showed evidence that regular physical activity during youth is related to lifestyle and health at adult age.

On the basis of the unfavorable trends with respect to risk factors for chronic diseases in the population and the knowledge that health promotional activities in youth may effect lifestyles, health and disease at adult age, it is important to know what the effects of a long-term at adolescent age started intervention are on risk factors for chronic diseases at adult age. The purpose of the present study, therefore, is to determine whether a series of medical check-ups and provisions of personal health information, beginning at age 13 years, has influenced biological risk factors for chronic diseases at age 32. It was hypothesized that the men and women who received more medical check-ups and personal health information would show a more positive 20-year change with respect to lifestyle and biological risk factors for chronic diseases relative to the men and women who did not receive these check-ups and information.

Methods

Population
This study is part of the Amsterdam Growth and Health Longitudinal Study (AGAHLS). This observational study started in 1977 with measurements in 420 boys and

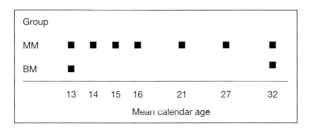

Fig. 1. Measurements in the Multi-Measurements Group (MM) and the Bi-Measurements Group (BM).

girls from two secondary schools. Participants from the first school had four annual measurements from ages 13 through 16 years. From 1981 to 1997, another four repeated measurements were completed at ages 21, 27, 29 and 32 years (so-called multi-measured group: MM). Participants from the second school were measured only two times, at ages 13 and 32 years (so-called bi-measured group: BM) [13]. The difference in number of measurements with health information between the MM and BM groups are given in figure 1.

Previous publications describe the design of AGAHLS extensively [14, 15]. As the AGAHLS was an observational study intending to describe the development of lifestyle, health and psychological variables, and the interrelations between these variables, there was no aim at intervention in this population. The contrast between the two groups was, therefore, never intended to result in differences in lifestyle or health between the groups. The second school was used to control for the possible confounding effects of repeated testing during adolescence [16]. In the present study, the difference in number of measurements and feedback about one's health is perceived as an 'intervention'. Here, it is investigated whether this unintended 'intervention' had any effect on lifestyles and biological risk factors for chronic diseases. Many participants did not attend all two (BM group) or eight (MM group) measurements. For the data of a participant to be included in the analyses, they had to be available as the pre- and post-'intervention' measurements (at ages 13 and 32 years). To receive maximal contrast, participants in the MM group needed to have attended at least four of the six in-between measurements. For the final data analysis a maximum of 164 MM group participants (92 females and 72 males), and a maximum of 113 BM group participants (54 females and 59 males) met these criteria.

'Intervention'

An overview of the measurements and health information given to the MM and BM group at the different ages is shown in table 1. Purposes of the lifestyle, health, fitness and psychological measurements were explained to the participants prior to their assessment. Immediate verbal feedback on the participants' performance on the fitness tests was given by the AGAHLS team members after the measurements, and additional information was given if requested by the participant. In addition to providing the personal result of, e.g., fitness, body composition, and blood pressure at the time of measurement, participants were also immediately informed about the changes with respect to their previous measurements.

Table 1. Overview of the measurements and information given to the two groups of participants at the different ages

Group	Age	Measurements and information given
Both groups	13	baseline measurement + brochure 'Growth and health 1' + 16 mm movie 'How healthy is growth?'
'Intervention' group only	14	measurement + brochure 'Growth and health 2'
	15	measurement + brochure 'Growth and health 3'
	16	measurement + brochure 'Growth and health 4'
	18	seminar with slide and VHS presentations of the 4-year longitudinal research results + book 'Growth and health of teenagers' + appendix with personal results
	21	measurement + book 'From teenager to adult' + appendix with personal results
	27	measurement + book '15 years Amsterdam growth and health study' + appendix with personal results
	29	measurement + book '17 years Amsterdam growth and health study' + appendix with personal results
Both groups	32	post-'intervention' measurement

Feedback in written form was given several months after the measurements. This included information about general results of the longitudinal study which entailed age- and gender-specific criteria and norm reference values to compare with, e.g. about obesity, hypertension, hypercholesterolemia, cigarette smoking, excess of energy intake, alcohol consumption, and hypoactivity. The reference values were retrieved from consensus-based documents published by leading health promotion organizations such as the American College of Sports Medicine, the Netherlands Olympic Committee/Netherlands Sports Federation, the Netherlands Heart Foundation, and the Dutch National Institute of Public Health and the Environment. An appendix with a selection of the individual results of the participant was added to the written feedback form.

If explicitly asked by the participant, participants were advised to change their lifestyle behavior. For instance, overweight participants with a high caloric intake and low physical activity were advised to change their energy balance by dieting and by becoming more active. In some other cases, participants with high blood pressure or high cholesterol levels were advised to visit their family doctor. Because the prevalence of hypertension, hypercholesterolemia and obesity became relatively high over the course of the study, 20–50% of the participants were advised to change their lifestyle. In an earlier publication [13], it was shown that participants with relatively 'poor' health at age 21 years had more positively changed their lifestyle at age 27 years, than the group that was in 'good' health (lower fat intake, higher physical activity level).

Measurements
Biological Risk Factors. Fat mass was estimated from the sum of four skinfolds (S4S) (biceps, triceps, subscapularis, crista iliaca) measured with a skinfold caliper

(Holtain, Van Rietschoten en Houwens, The Netherlands). The ratio between the subscapular and triceps skinfold (S/T) was calculated as a measure of fat distribution [17].

Blood pressure was measured indirectly with the participant seated in a chair, and with a standard pressure cuff (12-cm width) placed around the left upper arm. With a sphygmomanometer (Speidl-Keller, 2010, Franken & Itallie, The Netherlands) diastolic (phase V) blood pressure (DBP) and systolic blood pressure (SBP) were measured twice, and the lowest values of both DBP and SBP were recorded.

Blood cholesterol was determined by taking approximately 10 ml of venous blood from the vena antecubitus with a vacutainer (Becton, Dickinson, USA). The concentration of total serum cholesterol (TC) [18, 19], and high-density lipoprotein cholesterol (HDL) [20] were analyzed and the ratio between TC and HDL was calculated (TC/HDL). External quality control took place with reference samples from the WHO Lipid Standardization Laboratory, Atlanta, Ga., USA.

Cardiorespiratory fitness was operationalized as maximal oxygen uptake relative to body weight (VO_2max). VO_2max was measured directly with the participant running on a treadmill with a constant speed (8 km/h) and stepwise increasing slope till exhaustion. O_2 uptake and CO_2 production were measured continuously throughout the test using the open-circuit method. The volume of the expired air was measured with a 10-liter high-speed, low-resistance dry gas meter (Parkinson CD4) via a two-way low resistance breathing valve with a dead airspace of 35 ml. Expired air was analyzed for O_2 by a paramagnetic analyzer (Servomex) and for CO_2 by an infrared analyzer (Mijnhardt). The gas meter and the two analyzers were incorporated into a movable 19-inch unit (Ergoanalyzer, Mijnhardt, The Netherlands). This automated and computerized method was validated against the classical method of collecting expired air in Douglas bags and analyzing CO_2 and O_2 content with the Scholander technique [21].

Neuromotor fitness was operationalized by seven tests from the Motor Performance (MOPER) Fitness Test [22]. This MOPER test measures muscle strength, speed, and coordination. The scores of each test were ranked for men and women separately, the best scores giving the highest and the worst scores the lowest ranking. The rank numbers were then tallied and divided by the number of tests for each participant to obtain an overall ranking of neuromotor fitness [23].

Lifestyle Risk Factors. Daily physical activity was measured in the participants along the whole period of twenty years by means of a structured interview based on a physical activity questionnaire (PAQ) developed by Verschuur [24]. The PAQ consisted of questions about duration (minutes), frequency (per day, week) and intensity (metabolic rate) of all physical activities during the three months preceding the interview (PAQ was always conducted between February and June of each year of measurement). The following physical activities were included: organized and unorganized sports activities, leisure time activities, activities at school (physical education), at work and active transportation (cycling, walking, taking stairs).

Physical activities shorter than 5 min or with a metabolic intensity of less than 4 times resting metabolic rate (<4 MET) were not taken into consideration. All other physical activities were categorized in three intensity levels: light physical activity (4–7 MET), moderate physical activity (7–10 MET) and heavy physical activity (>10 MET) and expressed in minutes per week. Combining the three intensity levels, a weighted physical activity score was derived by multiplying the three intensity categories by their average MET-score: light by 5.5, moderate by 8.5 and heavy by 11; the weighted physical activity score was the sum of the minutes per week times the scores of the three intensity levels [25].

Detailed information about food consumption was obtained by means of a validated semi-structured cross-check dietary history interview concerning the frequency and amounts of intake and methods of preparation of food products, during the past month [26]. This cross-check dietary history interview was based on the assessment method developed by Burke [27] and adapted for the use in a teenage population [28–30]. The relative validity was checked with the 24-hour recall method [30]. The interview was done by one of the authors (G.B.P.) all over the 20 years in all participants to avoid observer error. The Dutch Food Composition Table [31] was used to calculate the intake amounts of several nutritional variables. In this chapter, the following variables are used:

Total energy intake per day expressed per kilogram bodyweight (En/kg).

Protein (total, vegetable, animal), fat (total, saturated fatty acids (SFA), mono unsaturated fatty acids (MUFA), polyunsaturated fatty acids (PUFA) and carbohydrate (total, mono/disaccharides, polysaccharides); intakes expressed as a percentage of total energy intake (En%).

Cholesterol, calcium, iron, thiamin, riboflavin, pyridoxine, retinol, vitamin E and ascorbic acid intake denoted in grams or milligrams per day.

Statistical Analysis

Baseline differences between dropouts and non-dropouts, and for the non-dropouts, between the 'intervention' and the BM group are tested with t tests for each of the nine outcome variables. The 20-year changes were calculated by subtracting the age 13 score from the score at age 32. Differences between the MM and BM group in these 20-year change scores were tested separately for men and women by multiple analysis of variance (MANOVA) for repeated measurements.

Results

Biological Risk Factors

Table 2 shows baseline data of the nine biological risk factors of the non-dropouts in the MM and BM group. In men, borderline significant healthier baseline values for the BM group were found for SFS and for SBP. In women, TC at baseline was borderline significantly worse in BM, while VO$_2$max was significantly worse in the MM group. For the other variables no significant baseline differences were found.

Table 3 shows the 20-year changes of the nine biological risk factors. In men, TC, TC/HDL, S4S, S/T, SBP, and DBP have increased, and HDL and VO$_2$max have decreased from age 13 to 32 years. On most of the seven MOPER tests, better values were attained at age 32 than at age 13 years. However, this increase in MOPER is solely due to the higher diversity in scores at age 32, causing a higher average ranking. In women, TC, HDL, S4S, S/T, and DBP increased, and VO$_2$max decreased over the 20 years of the study. No changes were seen in TC/HDL and SBP.

Table 2. Means and standard deviations (SD) of baseline values (age 13) of the nine biological risk factors for chronic diseases in men and women of the multi-measured (MM) and bi-measured (BM) group

| Factor | Unit | Men (n = 131) | | | | | Women (n = 146) | | | | |
| | | MM (n = 72) | | BM (n = 59) | | | MM (n = 92) | | BM (n = 54) | | |
		mean	SD	mean	SD	p value	mean	SD	mean	SD	p value
TC	mmol/l	4.5	0.7	4.4	0.7	0.94	4.4	0.7	4.6	0.8	0.05
HDL	mmol/l	1.5	0.3	1.5	0.3	0.88	1.4	0.3	1.5	0.3	0.36
TC/HDL		3.1	0.6	3.1	0.7	0.92	3.1	0.7	3.2	0.6	0.73
S4S	mm	29	12	25	8	0.06	37	14	36	10	0.77
S/T		0.71	0.19	0.72	0.19	0.85	0.71	0.18	0.68	0.20	0.32
SBP	mm Hg	125	9	121	9	0.04	124	10	125	8	0.73
DBP	mm Hg	74	8	75	7	0.33	77	7	75	8	0.10
MOPER		25.5	6.9	27.5	6.7	0.10	23.5	6.7	23.2	6.9	0.81
VO$_2$max	ml/kg/min	59.2	5.6	60.6	6.1	0.18	51.1	6.0	53.7	5.6	0.01

Table 3. Means and standard deviations (SD) of the 20-year change scores (age 32 minus age 13) of the nine biological risk factors for chronic diseases in men and women of the multi-measured (MM) and bi-measured (BM) group

| Factor | Unit | Men (n = 131) | | | | | Women (n = 146) | | | | |
| | | MM (n = 72) | | BM (n = 59) | | | MM (n = 92) | | BM (n = 54) | | |
		mean	SD	mean	SD	p value	mean	SD	mean	SD	p value
TC	mmol/l	0.5	0.7	0.6	0.9	0.64	0.4	0.7	0.4	0.8	0.99
HDL	mmol/l	−0.25	0.3	−0.32	0.3	0.17	0.15	0.3	0.13	0.3	0.74
TC/HDL		1.1	0.9	1.4	1.3	0.14	−0.0	0.6	0.1	0.7	0.36
S4S	mm	14	17	14	16	0.94	16	18	21	21	0.18
S/T		0.83	0.45	1.00	0.51	0.05	0.16	0.22	0.29	0.39	0.02
SBP	mm Hg	8	14	14	12	0.01	−1	10	1	10	0.16
DBP	mm Hg	11	10	10	10	0.75	6	10	7	10	0.72
MOPER		3.3	7.1	1.9	7.6	0.32	5.3	8.2	4.1	8.0	0.43
VO$_2$max	ml/kg/min	−13.4	7.6	−13.9	9.6	0.73	−11.8	7.1	−12.9	6.0	0.32

Table 4. Results of the MANOVA regarding the relationship between 20 years of health information with medical check-ups on the total physical activity of males and females; the activities are split in light, moderate and heavy intensities as well as a composite weighted score of the three intensities

Effects		Light physical activity	Moderate physical activity	Heavy physical activity	Total weighted physical activity
Group	males	=	=	=	=
	females	=	=	=	higher in BM
Time	males	⇑	⇓	⇓	⇓
	females	⇑	⇓	=	⇑
Time × group	males	=	+BM	=	=
	females	+BM	=	+BM	=

=: No significant difference (p > 0.05); ⇑: significant increase; ⇓: significant decrease; +BM: more favorable change in Bi-measured group.

In men, a borderline significant difference in the 20-year change was found for the S/T ratio, favoring the MM group with 0.17 (table 2). SBP in the BM group was 14 mm Hg higher at age 32 than at age 13. A significantly smaller, and thus healthier, increase of 8 mm Hg was seen in the MM group. In women, only one significant 'intervention' effect was seen. The 20-year change in the S/T ratio was 0.13 better in the MM than in the BM group. None of the other 20-year changes differed significantly between the two groups.

Physical Activity

The results of testing the levels of total physical activities with MANOVA are summarized in table 4. No effects (time × group interactions) of the health information were found: for total weighted physical activity the few statistically significant differences are in the not expected direction: males from the BM group show significant higher moderate total physical activities and females more light and heavy total physical activities compared to the MM group.

In table 4 apart from the 'intervention' effect (group X time) also the significant differences between MM and BM group (group effect) and age changes (time effect) are indicated: the differences in activities between males and females are not significant with one exception: the females from the BM group show more total weighted physical activities compared to the MM group. The age effects show that the males significantly decrease their total weighted physical activities. The females show an increase of light, decrease of moderate, no change in heavy physical activities and an increase in overall total weighted physical activities. No intervention effect was found for total physical

Table 5. Means and standard deviations (in parentheses) of energy and nutrient intake and p values of the 'intervention' effects

	Unit	Multi-measured group (MM)		Bi measured group (BM)		P-values Time*Group
		age 13	age 32	age 13	age 32	
Energy	kJ/kg	241.55 (67.57)	148.57 (32.43)	246.84 (60.26)	152.30 (42.24)	0.22
Nutrients						
Proteins	En%	14.04 (2.35)	15.55 (2.38)	14.56 (2.24)	15.26 (2.42)	0.06
Vegetable proteins	En%	5.14 (0.78)	5.71 (1.16)	5.31 (0.78)	5.64 (0.98)	0.23
Animal proteins	En%	8.94 (2.29)	9.75 (2.24)	9.26 (2.22)	9.54 (2.33)	0.19
Fat	En%	38.26 (4.78)	36.87 (5.61)	37.99 (4.40)	35.90 (5.07)	0.51
Saturated fatty acids	En%	12.26 (1.98)	11.20 (2.42)	12.41 (1.88)	11.21 (2.00)	0.97
Mono unsaturated fatty acids	En%	14.55 (2.29)	13.49 (2.38)	14.18 (2.20)	13.22 (2.27)	0.82
Poly unsaturated fatty acids	En%	5.79 (2.23)	6.04 (1.70)	5.65 (2.05)	5.48 (1.64)	0.13
Carbohydrates	En%	47.37 (4.58)	45.47 (5.57)	47.30 (4.61)	46.31 (5.07)	0.28
Mono-/disaccharides	En%	23.54 (4.34)	20.96 (5.08)	22.15 (4.40)	21.66 (4.70)	0.01
Polysaccharides	En%	23.86 (3.61)	24.39 (3.94)	25.17 (3.49)	24.57 (3.78)	0.07
Cholesterol	mg	316.41 (85.66)	272.33 (91.11)	310.03 (91.66)	289.88 (94.68)	0.13
Calcium	g	1.03 (0.39)	1.23 (0.41)	1.10 (0.45)	1.30 (0.57)	0.92
Iron	mg	11.30 (2.22)	13.48 (2.92)	11.51 (2.68)	13.95 (3.57)	0.91
Thiamin	mg	1.29 (0.40)	1.33 (0.35)	1.35 (0.47)	1.42 (0.46)	0.97
Riboflavin	mg	1.57 (0.52)	1.80 (0.50)	1.58 (0.47)	1.88 (0.74)	0.54
Pyridoxine	mg	1.62 (0.36)	1.93 (0.48)	1.70 (0.52)	2.02 (0.62)	0.72
Retinol	mg	1.15 (0.69)	0.91 (0.50)	1.11 (0.65)	0.89 (0.46)	0.86
Vitamin E	mg	15.95 (6.93)	14.53 (5.56)	15.35 (5.86)	14.27 (7.98)	0.91
Ascorbic acid	mg	116.23 (40.48)	139.56 (55.20)	114.70 (42.42)	154.87 (61.67)	0.06

activity, whereas unexpected more favorable changes of light, heavy (men), and moderately intense (women) physical activities were observed in BM group as compared with the MM group.

Dietary Intake

Means and standard deviations of energy intake and nutrients at age 13 and at age 32 are shown in table 5. A statistically significant 'intervention'-effect was found for the intake of mono-/disaccharides only. The average individual change of the intake of mono-/disaccharides (En%) was more favorable in the MM than in the BM group. Additionally, trends were found for protein intake (En%), polysaccharide intake (En%), cholesterol intake and the intake of ascorbic acid. The MM group tended to show (1) A larger increase of protein intake ($p < 0.07$); (2) A larger increase of polysaccharides intake ($p < 0.08$); (3) A larger decrease of cholesterol ($p < 0.09$), and (4) A smaller increase of the intake of ascorbic acid ($p < 0.07$) in comparison to the BM group.

Discussion

The purpose of this article was to describe the effects of six additional repeated medical check-ups with personal health information between age 13 and 32 on the development of biological and lifestyle risk factors. As the AGAHLS is an observational cohort study in an overall healthy population, these repeated medical check-ups and the information given were never intended to be an 'intervention'. But, the AGAHLS also consists of a group of men and women with measurements at age 13 and 32 only. In this article, this second group is seen as the BM group, and the group that received the six additional check-ups and feedbacks on their lifestyle and health is seen as the MM group.

Selective Dropout

Of the men and women with a baseline measurement at age 13 years, only 143 participants (34%) dropped out during the 20-year follow-up of the study. In both men and women the non-dropouts had better physical fitness at baseline. Cholesterol and body fat also showed healthier values in non-dropouts (significant in women). Several reasons for this selective dropout may be thought of. The measurements (such as the maximal running test on the treadmill) may have been so strenuous for those with low physical fitness that they no longer wanted to participate. Or, these participants dropped out because they did not want to be confronted with their poor physical fitness grade. These participants may also have stopped showing up at measurements because of feelings of shame due to their poor fitness. They possibly did not want to be confronted with the investigators or the (about seven)-other participants who were to be assessed on the same day. However, this is all just guess work. The only reasons for dropping out given by the participants were 'moved out of town' (only during the first four years of the study), 'no time', and 'no interest'. It is not expected that chronic disease or mortality related to the factors under study here have caused dropout.

'Intervention' Effects

Biological Risk Factors. Of the nine biological risk factors for chronic diseases, only the changes in S/T favored the MM group in both men and women. That an 'intervention' effect was found especially for this factor was not expected, as one has probably less personal control over S/T than over each of the other eight risk factors. Therefore, a type I error is expected. Bouchard [32] has shown in a study of monozygotic twins that body fat distribution can be changed by a manipulation of energy balance. However, the 'intervention' in our study has not shown to lead to a healthier energy balance. Also, an effect of a healthier energy balance would have been more plausible for SFS than for S/T.

The other risk factor for which a significant 'intervention' effect was found was SBP in men. It is possible that SBP in the MM group has increased less because of the discovery of high BP in some of the participants at 1 of the 6 in-between measurements. In such a case, advice was given to visit the family doctor, who in turn may have advised on improving lifestyle or may have prescribed medication to lower BP. However, the effect of medication appears negligible as only one of the men in the MM group reported taking such medication. Also, medication or a change of lifestyle would probably affect DBP in the same direction, whereas for DBP a slight trend in the opposite direction was found. However, this opposite result may be due to the low reproducibility of DBP in this longitudinal study [14].

A more plausible explanation of the observed 'intervention' effect on SBP is regression to the mean. At baseline, despite the fact that the same experienced tester (H.K.) performed the measurements in both groups, SBP was significantly lower in the BM group than in the MM group. If this difference at baseline was a systematic measurement error, it would explain more than half of the 'intervention' effect. If the analysis was performed with correcting for SBP at baseline, the difference in SBP increase between the two groups was no longer significant ($p = 0.10$). Another explanation for the found difference in SBP change may be that the men in the MM group may have become more acquainted with the measurements as compared with the men in the BM group resulting in the slightly higher SBP at age 32 in the BM group.

The development of the other seven risk factors did not significantly differ between the MM and BM group. It is possible that the participants in the MM group had in fact changed their lifestyle in a healthier direction than the BM group, but that this difference had not translated (yet) into measurable differences in the biological risk factors. The AGAHLS recently has presented arguments for this possibility by showing that dramatic decreases in physical activity during the first four years of the study and continuing excessive protein and fat intake and too low carbohydrate intake have not immediately resulted in deteriorated biological factors [33, 34].

Physical Activity. Total weighted physical activity scores did not decrease less in the MM group compared to the BM group in both males and females. The unexpected result that the BM group decreased their light (females) physical activity, moderate (males) physical activity and heavy (females) physical activity less than the MM group suggest negative effects of the medical checkups with health information, which seems difficult to explain. It may be caused by a confounding effect that can occur in longitudinal research and that is inevitably connected with repeated measurements. During the adolescent

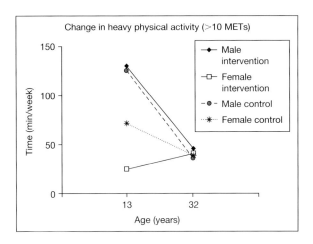

Fig. 2. MET scores of heavy (>10) physical activities in males and females at 13 and 33 years of age in the BM (control) and MM (intervention) groups.

period in boys and girls the total time per week spent doing physical activities decreased more in the group that had four annual measurements than in the group that was measured only once in the four years. This was interpreted as a negative testing effect rather than as an actual decline in the amount of physical activity: with repeated activity interviews the participants in the MM group on average, may be inclined to underreporting their physical activities [35].

In line with this finding over the first 4 years, it is possible that at age 32 years, the females in the MM group underreported their heavy physical activity levels more as compared with the BM group (fig. 2).

It is difficult to compare the results of the present study with other health-promotional studies, because the interventions differ remarkably between studies. The present study used only a health informational approach and not a health educational approach. Moreover, the health information was only given to the participants on a face to face basis. Pate et al. [36] stated that in order to be effective the health educational intervention needs to be given at different levels: not only to individuals but also to public health agencies, health professionals, communities, educators and families.

Dietary Intake. Very few 'intervention' effects concerning dietary intake were found. Some evidence was found for a different development of mono- and disaccharides intake over time: the MM group showed a stronger decrease through time than the BM group. It is important to note, however, that after application of the Holm correction [37], the 'intervention' effect should not be considered as statistically significant. Furthermore, in both groups the average

Table 6. Proportions of the participants in the multi-measured group (MM) and bi-measured group (BM), of which the dietary intake at age 32 years was not in accordance with the recommendations of the Netherlands Nutrition Council (1989) and the p values of the χ^2 test

	MMG %	BMG %	p (χ^2 test)
Proportions above the maximally recommended amounts			
Energy[1]	59	56	0.67
Proteins	94	94	0.86
Animal proteins	100	100	_[2]
Fat	62	56	0.30
Saturated fatty acids	94	98	0.88
Mono-/disaccharides	18	22	0.45
Carbohydrates	97	94	0.33
Calcium	9	10	0.82
Iron[1]	46	42	0.59
Thiamin[1]	18	17	0.21
Riboflavin[1]	26	33	0.19
Pyridoxine[1]	4	4	0.95
Retinol[1]	40	56	0.46
Ascorbic acid	4	10	0.07

[1]Proportions are based on gender-specific recommendations.
[2]No outcome, since all values were above the recommendations.

intake of mono- and disaccharides was below the maximally recommended amounts anyway, and thus should not be considered as unhealthy. In addition, the proportions of participants at age 32 that had a diet that was not in accordance with the Dutch recommendations did not differ between the MM and the BM groups for energy or for any of the nutrients. An exception may be the trend concerning ascorbic acid intake, which is in favor of the MM group (table 6). In sum, these results do not reflect a clear-cut positive effect of repeated measurements and health information, resulting in healthier dietary intake.

Small Contrast. A more likely reason as to why the medical check-ups with personal health information did not alter the biologic and lifestyle risk factors may be that the difference between the MM group and BM group in the number of measurements attended was too small. Most participants in the MM group had attended all six additional measurements. However, our subjective criterion of a contrast of at least four measurements may have resulted in little effect in many participants, especially in view of the long period of time over which these few 'intervention' measurements with feedback on health took place. Particularly when a participant in the MM group missed the last 'intervention' measurement at the age of 29 years, a possible health effect of the five measurements taken from age 14 until 27 years may have completely faded at age 32. Lastly there may have been other aspects underlying the too small contrast between the groups. Mass media health and lifestyle promotions in the community during the study period may have influenced both groups to such a degree that a ceiling effect made the here studied 'intervention' no longer effective. It is also possible that an 'intervention' such as the present one had no effect because of the relatively young and healthy population. If the same kind of 'intervention' would have been executed in an older population, where chronic diseases are more prevalent, it might have been effective. However, most studies on adults have shown no beneficial effect on fitness either [38].

The repeated medical check-ups with personal health information in the present study did not involve a health education [34]. Therefore, the absence in this study of a theoretically-based intervention, like Prochaska's model of the stages of change [10] may be related to the absence of a positive effect of the 'intervention'. Recently, Simons-Morton [39] reported on the effects of physical activity counseling interventions with regard to improving cardiorespiratory fitness. Thus, a reason for not finding significant 'intervention' effects here may be that the information in the present study was given solely to the participants. Moreover, the health information was only aiming at knowledge, and not at other relevant determinants such as attitudes and social support [11].

Summary and Conclusion

The purpose of this study was to determine the effects of repeated medical check-ups with health information over a period of 20 years on biological and lifestyle risk factors for chronic diseases using data from the Amsterdam Growth and Health Longitudinal Study. Significant 'intervention' effects were found for two of the nine biological risk factors, and one of the twenty dietary risk factors only. These are probably type I errors. Contrary to the hypothesis that repeated health information and medical check-ups should increase the physical activity levels, the males and females from the BM group showed a higher increase (or a lower decrease) over the 20-year period in both sports and total physical activities compared to the MM group. Reasons for the absence of a clear positive effect of this health informational 'intervention' may be found in the low contrast between the groups over the 20 years of the study, and in the absence of an intention and of effort to improve lifestyle and health.

References

1   Bouchard C, Malina RM, Perusse L (eds): Genetics of Fitness and Physical Performance. Champaign, Human Kinetics, 1997.

2   Blair SN, Kohl HW, Paffenbarger RS, Clark DG, Cooper KH, Gibbons LW: Physical fitness and all cause mortality: A prospective study of healthy men and women. JAMA 1989;262:2395–2401.

3   Ruwaard D, Kramers PGN (eds): Public Health Exploration of the Future [in Dutch: Volksgezondheid Toekomst Verkenning 1997, de som der delen]. Rijksinstituut voor Volksgezondheid en Milieu. Utrecht, Elsevier/De Tijdstroom, 1997.

4   Caspersen CJ: Physical activity epidemiology, concepts, methods and applications to exercise science. Exerc Sport Sci Rev 1989;17:423–473.

5   Kok GJ: Theories about influencing behavior [in Dutch: Theorieën over gedragsbeïnvloeding]; in Damoiseaux V, Gerards FM, Kok GJ, Nijhuis F (eds): Gezondheidsvoorlichting en –opvoeding. Van analyse tot effecten. Assen/Maastricht, Van Gorcum, 1987, pp 35–77.

6   Dishman RK, Sallis JF: Determinants and interventions for physical activity and exercise; in Bouchard C, Shephard RJ, Stephens T (eds): Physical Activity, Fitness and Health: International Proceedings and Consensus Statement. Champaign, Human Kinetics, 1994, pp 214–238.

7   Dishman RK: Determinants of participation in physical activity; in Bouchard C, Shephard RJ, Stephens T, Sutton JR, McPherson BD (eds): Exercise, Fitness and Health: A Consensus of Current Knowledge. Champaign, Human Kinetics, 1990, pp 75–101.

8   Ajzen I, Fishbein M: Understanding Attitudes and Predicting Social Behavior. Englewood Cliffs, Prentice Hall, 1980.

9   Janz NK, Becker MH: The health belief model. Health Edu Q 1984;11:1–47.

10 Prochaska JD, Diclemente CC, Norcross JC: In search of how people change: Applications to addictive behaviors. Am Psychol 1992;47:1102–1114.

11 Dishman RK (ed): Exercise Adherence: Its Impact on Public Health. Champaign, Human Kinetics 1988.

12 Kuh DJ, Cooper C: Physical activity at 36 years: Patterns and childhood predictors in a longitudinal study. J Epidemiol Community Health 1992;46,2:114–119.

13 Kemper HCG, van Mechelen W, Post GB, Snel J, Twisk JWR, van Lenthe FJ, Welten DC: The Amsterdam Growth and Health Longitudinal Study, the past (1976–1996) and future (1997–?). Int J Sports Med 1997;18(suppl 3):140–150.

14 Kemper HCG (ed): Growth, health and fitness of teenagers, longitudinal research in international perspective. Med Sport Sci. Basel, Karger, 1985, vol 20.

15 Kemper HCG (ed): The Amsterdam Growth Study, a longitudinal analysis of health, fitness, and lifestyle. HK Sport Science Monograph Series. Champaign, Human Kinetics, 1995, vol 6.

16 Kemper HCG, van 't Hof MA: Design of a multiple longitudinal study of growth and health of teenagers. Eur J Pediatr 1978;129:147–155.

17 van Lenthe FJ, Snel J, Twisk JWR, van Mechelen W, Kemper HCG: Coping, personality and the development of a central pattern of body fat from youth into adulthood: The Amsterdam Growth and Health Longitudinal Study. Int J Obes 1998;22:861–868.

18 Huang TC, Chen CP, Wefler V, Raftery A: A stable reagent for the Lieberman-Buchard reaction. Anal Chem 1961;33:1405–1407.

19 Abell LL, Levy BB, Brody BB, Kendall FE: Simplified method for the estimation of total cholesterol in serum and demonstration of its specificity. J Biol Chem 1952;195:357–366.

20 Burnstein M, Samaille J: Sur un dosage rapide du cholesterol lie aux alpha- et aux betalipoproteinen du serum. Clin Chim Acta 1960;5:609–611.

21 Kemper HCG, Binkhorst RA, Verschuur R, Vissers ACA: Reliability of the Ergoanalyzer. J Cardiovasc Technol 1976;4:27–30.

22 Kemper HCG, Verschuur R, Schalekamp H, Storm-van Essen L: The MOPER-Fitness-Test II – An allometric approach to the arrangement of normscales. Proceedings of ICPFR 1978. S Afr J Res Sport Phys Educ Recreation 1979;2:94–99.

23 Twisk JWR, Staal BJ, Brinkman MN, Kemper HCG, van Mechelen W: Tracking of lung function parameters and the longitudinal relationship with lifestyle, Eur Respir J 1998;12:627–634.

24 Verschuur R: Daily physical activity and health: Longitudinal changes during the teenage period; thesis, Universiteit van Amsterdam. Haarlem, De Vrieseborch, 1987.
25 Montoye HJ, Kemper HCG, Saris WHM, Washburn RA: Measuring Physical Activity and Energy Expenditure. Champaign, Human Kinetics, 1996.
26 Post GB: Nutrition in adolescence. a longitudinal study in dietary patterns from teenager to adult; thesis, University of Wageningen. Haarlem, De Vrieseborch, 1989.
27 Burke BS: The dietary history as a tool in research. J Am Diet Assoc 1947;23:1041–1046.
28 Marr JW: Individual dietary surveys. Wld Rev Nutr Diet. Basel, Karger, 1971, vol 13, pp 105–164.
29 Beal VA: The nutritional history in longitudinal research. J Am Diet Assoc 1967;51:426–432.
30 Cameron ME, van Staveren WA (eds): Manual on Methodology for Food Consumption Studies. Oxford, Oxford University Press, 1988.
31 'Nederlandse Voedingsstoffen (NEVO)-tabel' (Dutch Food Composition Table): Stichting NEVO, Voorlichtingsbureau voor de voeding, 1989.
32 Bouchard C: Inheritance of fat distribution; in Bouchard C, Johnston FE (eds): Fat Distribution during Growth and Later Health Outcomes. New York, Liss, 1988, pp 103–125.
33 Post GB, de Vente W, Kemper HCG, Twisk JWR: Longitudinal trends in and tracking of energy and nutrient intake over 20 years on a Dutch cohort of men and women between 13 and 33 years of age: The Amsterdam growth and health longitudinal study. Br J Nutr 2001;85:375–385.
34 van Mechelen W, Twisk JWR, Post GB, Snel J, Kemper HCG: Physical activity of young people: The Amsterdam Growth and Health Study. Med Sci Sports Exerc 2000;32:1610–1616.
35 Kemper HCG, Dekker HJP, Ootjers MG, Post GB, Ritmeester J-W, Snel J, Splinter P, Storm-van Essen L, Verschuur R: Growth and health of teenagers in the Netherlands: Survey of Multidisciplinary Longitudinals Studies and comparison to recent results of a Dutch study. Int J Sports Med 1983;4:202–214.
36 Pate RR, Pratt M, Blair SN, Haskell WL, Macera CA, Bouchard C, Buchner D, Ettinger W, Heath GW, King AC, Kriska AC, Leon AS, Marcus BH, Morris J, Paffenbarger RS, Patrick K, Polluck ML, Rippe JM, Sallis J, Wilmore JH: Physical activity and public health. A recommendation from the Centers for Disease Control and Prevention and the American College of Sports Medicine. JAMA 1995;273:402–407.
37 Holm SA: A simple sequentially rejective multiple test procedure. Scand J Stat 1979;6:65–70.
38 Bruce RA, De Roonen TA, Hossack KF: Pilot study examining the motivational effects of maximal exercise testing to modify risk factors and health habits. Cardiology 1980;2:111–119.
39 Simons-Morton DG: Effects of physical activity counseling in primary care. JAMA 2001;286:677–687.

Prof. Dr. Han C.G. Kemper
AGAHLS Research Group, Institute for Research in Extramural Medicine
VU University Medical Center
Van der Boechorststraat 7, NL–1081 BT Amsterdam (The Netherlands)
Tel. +31 20 4448407, Fax +31 20 4446775, E-Mail hcg.kemper.emgo@med.vu.nl

Kemper HCG (ed): Amsterdam Growth and Health Longitudinal Study.
Med Sport Sci. Basel, Karger, 2004, vol 47, pp 183–193

....

Appendix: Publications from the Amsterdam Growth and Health Longitudinal Study

References

1   Ariens GAM, van Mechelen W, Kemper HCG, Twisk JWR: The longitudinal development of running economy in males and females aged between 13 and 27 years: The Amsterdam Growth and Health Study. Eur J Appl Physiol Occup Physiol 1997;76:214–220.
2   Bakker I, Kemper HCG, Twisk JWR, van Mechelen W: Bone mass at adult age is in different ways positively related to physical activity during adolescence and adulthood (abstract). Osteoporos Int 2000;11:S59.
3   Bakker I: Affectors of the adult lumbar bone: genetics, body composition and lifestyle; Diss. Vrije Universiteit, GIB publ. No. 12, Amsterdam, 2003.
4   Bakker I, Twisk JWR, van Mechelen W, Mensink GBM, Kemper HCG: Computerization of a dietary history interview in a running cohort; evaluation within the Amsterdam Growth and Health Longitudinal Study. Eur J Clin Nutr 2003;57:394–404.
5   Bakker I, Twisk JWR, van Mechelen W, Roos JC, Kemper HCG: Ten-year longitudinal relationship between physical activity and lumbar bone mass in (young) adults. J Bone Miner Res 2003; 18:325–332.
6   Bakker I, Twisk JWR, van Mechelen W, Kemper HCG: Fat-free body mass is the most important body composition determinant of 10-yr longitudinal development of lumbar bone in adult men and women. J Clin Endocrinol Metab 2003;88:2607–2613.
7   Bernaards CM: Smoking and health from adolescence into adulthood, results from the Amsterdam Growth and Health Longitudinal Study; Diss. Vrije Universiteit, GIB publ. No. 11, Amsterdam, 2003.
8   Bernaards CM, Kemper HCG, Twisk JWR, van Mechelen W, Snel J: Smoking behaviour and biological maturation in males and females: A 20-year longitudinal study. Analysis of data from the Amsterdam Growth and Health Longitudinal Study. Ann Hum Biol 2001;28:634–648.
9   Bernaards CM, Twisk JWR, Snel J, van Mechelen W, Kemper HCG: Is calculating pack-years retrospectively a valid method to estimate life-time tobacco smoking? A comparison between prospectively calculated pack-years and retrospectively calculated pack-years. Addiction 2001;96: 1653–1661.
10 Bernaards CM, Twisk JWR, van Mechelen W, Snel J, Kemper HCG: A longitudinal study on smoking in relationship to fitness and heart rate response. Med Sci Sports Exerc 2003;35: 793–800.
11 de Vente W, Post GB, Twisk JWR, Kemper HCG, van Mechelen W: Effects of health measurements and health information in youth and young adulthood in dietary intake – 20-y study results from the Amsterdam Growth and Health Longitudinal Study. Eur J Clin Nutr 2001;55: 819–823.
12 Dekker HJ, Ritmeester JW, Snel J: Personality traits and school attitude; in Kemper HCG (ed): Growth, Health and Fitness of Teenagers: Longitudinal Research in International Perspective. Basel, Karger, 1985, pp 137–147.

13   Dekker HJ, Ritmeester JW, Snel J: Psychosocial methods; in Kemper HCG (ed): Growth, Health and Fitness of Teenagers: Longitudinal Research in International Perspective. Basel, Karger, 1985, pp 47–52.
14   Ferreira I, Twisk JWR, van Mechelen W, Kemper HCG, Stehouwer CDA: Impact of changes in cardiorespiratory fitness from adolescence to adulthood on carotid atherosclerosis and large-artery stiffness: The Amsterdam Growth and Health Longitudinal Study. Circulation 2003;107:37.
15   Ferreira I, Twisk JWR, van Mechelen W, Kemper HCG, Stehouwer CDA: Current and adolescent levels of cardiopulmonary fitness are related to large artery properties at age 36: The Amsterdam Growth and Health Longitudinal Study. Eur J Clin Invest 2002;32:723–731.
16   Ferreira I, Twisk JWR, Stehouwer CDA, van Mechelen W, Kemper HCG: Longitudinal changes in $\dot{V}o_2$ max: associations with carotid intima-media thickness and arterial stifness. Med Sci Sports Exerc. Basel, Karger, 2003, vol 35, pp 1670–1678.
17   Groothausen J, Siemer H, Kemper HCG, Twisk JWR, Welten DC: Influence of peak strain on lumbar bone mineral density: An analysis of 15-year physical activity in young males and females. Pediatric Exerc Sci 1997;9:159–173.
18   Kemper HCG: Are there differences between early and late maturers in body composition and physical performances when they are adult? The Amsterdam Growth and Health Study; in Rohmert W, Wenzel HG (eds): Aspekte der Leistungsfähigteit (Different Aspects of Performance). Frankfurt am Main, Lange, 1989, pp 90–97.
19   Kemper HCG: Cardiovascular health and physical activity in youth: Results from the Amsterdam Growth and Health Study; in Smodis I, Szabó T, Mészáros J (eds): International Round Table Conference on Sports Physiology. Budapest, 1992, pp 37–46.
20   Kemper HCG: Childhood activity and physical development (abstract). Ann Hum Biol 1991;18:551–552.
21   Kemper HCG: Growth, health and fitness of teenagers. Longitudinal research in international perspective; in Kemper HCG (ed): Growth, Health and Fitness of Teenagers: Longitudinal Research in International Perspective. Basel, Karger, 1985.
22   Kemper HCG: Health and fitness of Dutch teenagers, a review; in Day JAP (ed): Proceedings of the Olympic Scientific Congress. Champaign, Human Kinetics, 1986, pp 61–80.
23   Kemper HCG: How important is physical activity for the development of aerobic power in youth? Sci Motricité 1992;17:44–50.
24   Kemper HCG: Introduction to the Amsterdam Growth and Health Study; in Kemper HCG (ed): The Amsterdam Growth Study: A Longitudinal Analysis of Health, Fitness and Lifestyle. Champaign, Human Kinetics, 1995, pp 1–5.
25   Kemper HCG: Is leg muscle mass decisive in reaching a plateau in oxygen uptake during maximal treadmill running? Analysis of data from the Amsterdam Growth and Health Study. Am J Hum Biol 1994;6:437–444.
26   Kemper HCG: Literature survey of longitudinal growth research; in Kemper HCG (ed): Growth, Health and Fitness of Teenagers: Longitudinal Research in International Perspective. Basel, Karger, 1985, pp 1–11.
27   Kemper HCG: Longitudinal research: It is magic! Int J Sports Med 1997;18:S139.
28   Kemper HCG: Longitudinal studies during growth and training: Importance and principles; in Oded Bar-Or (ed): The Child and Adolescent Athlete. Oxford, Blackwell Science, 1996, VI of The Encyclopaedia of Sports Medicine, pp 317–634.
29   Kemper HCG: Longitudinal studies of health and fitness of teenagers and the interaction with sports activity. Med Sport 1999;3:85–102.
30   Kemper HCG: Longitudinal studies on the development of health and fitness and the interaction with physical activity of teenagers. Pediatrician 1986;13:52–59.
31   Kemper HCG: The natural history of physical activity and aerobic fitness in teenagers; in Dishman RK (ed): Advances in Exercise Adherence. Champaign, Human Kinetics, 1994, pp 293–318.
32   Kemper HCG: Prevalence of risk-indicators for cardiovascular diseases in teenagers in the Netherlands. Tijdschr Soc Geneesk 1982;60:597–599.
33   Kemper HCG: Project growth and health of teenagers, a mixed longitudinal study (The Netherlands); in Mednick SA, Baert AE (eds): Prospective Longitudinal Research: An Empirical

Basis for the Primary Prevention of Psychosocial Disorders. Oxford, Oxford University Press, 1981, pp 109–111.

34 Kemper HCG: Relationship of physical activity and fitness in youth. Sci Sports 2001;16:7–11.

35 Kemper HCG: Role of the pediatric exercise scientist in physical education, sports training and physiotherapy. Int J Sports Med 2000;21:S118–S123.

36 Kemper HCG: Skeletal development in children and adolescents and the relations with physical activity; in Froberg H, Lammert O, St Hansem H, Blimkie CJR (eds): Proceedings of the International Symposium of Pediatric Work Physiology. Children and Exercise XVIII. Odense, Odense University Press, 1998, pp 139–160.

37 Kemper HCG: Sources of variation in longitudinal assessment of maximal aerobic power in teenage boys and girls: The Amsterdam Growth and Health Study. Hum Biol 1991;63:533–557.

38 Kemper HCG, Bakker I, Twisk JWR, van Mechelen W: Validation of a physical activity questionnaire to measure the effect of mechanical strain on bone mass. Bone 2002;30:799–804.

39 Kemper HCG, Bakker I, van Mechelen W, Post GB, Twisk JWR: Lumbar bone mass of adult males and females is positively related to physical activity patterns in adolescence and young adulthood. Medicina Sportiva 2001;5:E43–E47.

40 Kemper HCG, Brouwer N, Ootjers MG, Post GB, Ritmeester JW, Snel J, Splinter PG, Storm-van Essen L, Verschuur R: Wachstum und gesundheit von jugendlichen in den Niederlanden, eine interdisziplinaire untersuchung. Sportwissenschaft 1987;17:394–410.

41 Kemper HCG, de Vente W, van Mechelen W, Twisk JWR: Adolescent motor skill and performance: Is physical activity in adolescence related to adult physical fitness? Am J Hum Biol 2001; 13:180–189.

42 Kemper HCG, Dekker HJ, Ootjers MG, Post GB, Ritmeester JW, Snel J, Splinter PG, Storm-van Essen L, Verschuur R: How healthy are Dutch teenagers?; in Kemper HCG (ed): Growth, Health and Fitness of Teenagers: Longitudinal Research in International Perspective. Basel, Karger, 1985, pp 187–192.

43 Kemper HCG, Dekker HJ, Ootjers MG, Post GB, Ritmeester JW, Snel J, Splinter PG, Storm-van Essen L, Verschuur R: The problems of analyzing longitudinal data from the study 'growth and health of teenagers'; in Binkhorst RA, Kemper HCG, Saris WH (eds): Proceedings of the XIth International Symposium of Pediatric Work Physiology. Children and Exercise XI; Papendal, The Netherlands. Champaign, Human Kinetics, 1985, pp 233–252.

44 Kemper HCG, Dekker HJ, Ootjers MG, Post GB, Snel J, Splinter PG, Storm-van Essen L, Verschuur R: Growth and health of teenagers in the Netherlands: Survey of multidisciplinary longitudinal studies and comparison to recent results of a Dutch study. Int J Sports Med 1983;4:202–214.

45 Kemper HCG, Koppes LLJ, de Vente W, van Lenthe FJ, van Mechelen W, Twisk JWR, Post GB: Effects of health information in youth and young adulthood on risk factors for chronic diseases – 20-year study results from the Amsterdam Growth and Health Longitudinal Study. Prev Med 2002;35:533–539.

46 Kemper HCG, Niemeijer CJ, Martins Dias XJ, van Dieën JH: Is there a relationship between shrinkage and bone mineral density of the lumbar soine in healthy 27-year-old males and females: Papers on Anthropology VIII. Tartu, University of Tartu, 1999, pp 71–88.

47 Kemper HCG, Post GB, Twisk JWR: Rate of maturation during the teenage years: Nutrient intake and physical activity between ages 12 and 22. Int J Sport Nutr 1997;7:229–240.

48 Kemper HCG, Post GB, Twisk JWR, van Mechelen W: Lifestyle and obesity in adolescence and young adulthood: Results from the Amsterdam Growth And Health Longitudinal Study (AGAHLS). Int J Obes Relat Metab Disord 1999;23:S34–S40.

49 Kemper HCG, Post GB, Welten DC, van Mechelen W, Twisk JWR: What are the effects of calcium intake on bone health in young males and females: Analysis of data from the Amsterdam Growth and Health Longitudinal Study (AGAHLS). Acta Kinesiol Univ Tartuensis 2001;6:8–10.

50 Kemper HCG, Snel J, Verschuur R, Storm-van Essen L: Tracking of health and risk indicators of cardiovascular diseases from teenager to adult: Amsterdam Growth and Health Study. Prev Med 1990;19:642–655.

51 Kemper HCG, Storm-van Essen L, Splinter PG: Procedures and subjects; in Kemper HCG (ed): Growth, Health and Fitness of Teenagers: Longitudinal Research in International Perspective. Basel, Karger, 1985, pp 26–34.

52   Kemper HCG, Storm-van Essen L, van 't Hof MA: Measurement of growth velocity and peak height velocity in teenagers; in Borms J, Hauspie R, Sand A, Suzanne C, Hebbelinck M (eds): Prospective Longitudinal Research: An Empirical Basis for the Primary Prevention of Psychosocial Disorders. New York, Plenum, 1984, pp 311–318.

53   Kemper HCG, Storm-van Essen L, Verschuur R: Height velocity in a group of teenage boys. Ann Hum Biol 1985;12:545–349.

54   Kemper HCG, Storm-van Essen L, Verschuur R: Height, weight and height velocity; in Kemper HCG (ed): Growth, Health and Fitness of Teenagers: Longitudinal Research in International Perspective. Basel, Karger, 1985, pp 66–80.

55   Kemper HCG, Storm-van Essen L, Verschuur R: Tracking of risk indicators for coronary heart diseases from teenager to adult: The Amsterdam Growth and Health Study; in Oseid S, Carlsen K (eds): Proceedings of the International Symposium of Pediatric Work Physiology. Children and Exercise XIII; Hurdal, Norway. Champaign, Human Kinetics, 1989, pp 235–245.

56   Kemper HCG, Twisk JWR, Koppes LLJ, van Mechelen W, Post GB: A 15-year physical activity pattern is positively related to aerobic fitness in young males and females (13–27 years). Eur J Appl Physiol 2001;84:395–402.

57   Kemper HCG, Twisk JWR, van Mechelen W, Post GB, Roos JC, Lips P: A fifteen-year longitudinal study in young adults on the relation of physical activity and fitness with the development of the bone mass: The Amsterdam Growth and Health Longitudinal Study. Bone 2000;27: 847–853.

58   Kemper HCG, van Mechelen W: Methods of measurements used in the longitudinal study; in Kemper HCG (ed): The Amsterdam Growth Study: A Longitudinal Analyses of Health, Fitness and Lifestyle. Champaign, Human Kinetics, 1995, pp 17–28.

59   Kemper HCG, van Mechelen W: Physical fitness and the relationship to physical activity; in Kemper HCG (ed): The Amsterdam Growth Study: A Longitudinal Analyses of Health, Fitness and Lifestyle. Champaign, Human Kinetics, 1995, pp 174–188.

60   Kemper HCG, van Mechelen W, Post GB, Snel J, Twisk JWR, Buitendijk I, Jekel J, Lips P, Teule GJJ: The Amsterdam Growth and Health Study: A 15 years follow-up of male and female from age 13–27; in Coudert J, van Praagh E (eds): Proceedings of the XVIth International Congress on Pediatric Work Physiology. Children and Exercise XVI; Saint-Sauves d'Auvergne, France. Paris, Masson, 1992, pp 209–212.

61   Kemper HCG, van Mechelen W, Post GB, Snel J, Twisk JWR, van Lenthe FJ, Welten DC: The Amsterdam Growth and Health Longitudinal Study: The past (1976–1996) and future (1997–?). Int J Sports Med 1997;18:S140–S150.

62   Kemper HCG, van Mechelen W, Post GB, Twisk JWR, Bakker I: Peak bone mass of males and females at adult age is positively related to physical activity in adolescence (abstract). Children's Bone Health 1999;Osteoporosis International:41.

63   Kemper HCG, van Mechelen W, Post GB, Twisk JWR, de Vente W: Longitudinal relationship between the development of body fat mass in adolescent males and females and their eating and activity pattern; in Jürimäe T, Hills AP (eds): Body Composition Assessment in Children and Adolescents. Basel, Karger, 2001, vol 44, pp 155–167.

64   Kemper HCG, van Mechelen W, Twisk JWR: Interaction of physical-activity and age on the maximal aerobic power of 13-year-old to 27-year-old males and females (abstract). J Physiol Lond 1994;479:P50.

65   Kemper HCG, van Praagh E: Croissance et évolution de la performance motrice chez les adolescents. Rev Educ Phys Sport 1986;197:16–19.

66   Kemper HCG, van 't Hof MA: Design of a multiple longitudinal study of growth and health in teenagers. Eur J Pediatr 1978;129:147–155.

67   Kemper HCG, van 't Hof MA: Eine Gemischte Laengsschnittuntersuchung zur Beschreibung von Wachstum und Gesundheit bei Jugendlichen in den Niederlanden; in Willimczik K, Grosser M (eds): Die Motorische Entwicklung im Kindes- und Jungendalter. Schorndorf, Hofmann, 1979, pp 119–132.

68   Kemper HCG, van 't Hof MA: Measurement of aerobic power in teenagers; in Morehouse C (ed): Proceedings of the International Symposium of Pediatric Work Physiology. Children and Exercise IX; Marstand, Sweden. Baltimore, University Park Press, 1980, pp 55–63.

69   Kemper HCG, van Zundert A: The role of leg muscle mass in reaching a levelling-off in oxygen uptake during maximal treadmill running in male and female adolescents; in Frenkl R, Szmodis I (eds): Proceedings of the International Symposium on Pediatric Work Physiology. Children and Exercise XV; Seregélyes, Hungary. Budapest, National Institute of Health Promotion (NEVI), 1991, pp 65–73.

70   Kemper HCG, van Zundert A, Verschuur R: Effects of rate of maturation on body composition and physical performance of young men and females: The Amsterdam Growth and Health Study; in Beunen G, Ghesquiere J, Reijbrouck T, Claessens AL (eds): Proceedings of the International Symposium on Pediatric Work Physiology. Children and Exercise XIV; Leuven, Belgium. Stuttgart, Enke, 1990, pp 11–19.

71   Kemper HCG, vd Bom C, Dekker HJ, Ootjers MG, Post GB, Snel J, Splinter PG, Storm-van Essen L, Verschuur R: A multiple longitudinal study of growth and health in teenagers in The Netherlands (abstract). Int J Sports Med 1982;3:182.

72   Kemper HCG, Vergouwe Y, Twisk JWR: Is there an association between biological maturation during adolescence and cardiovascular disease risk factors in adulthood? Results from the Amsterdam Growth and Health Longitudinal Study. Acta Acad Olymp Eston 2000;7:90–106.

73   Kemper HCG, Verhagen EALM, Milo D, Post GB, van Lenthe FJ, van Mechelen W, Twisk JWR, de Vente W: Effects of health information in youth on adult physical activity: 20-year study results from the Amsterdam Growth and Health Longitudinal Study. Am J Hum Biol 2002;14: 448–456.

74   Kemper HCG, Verschuur R: Biological development; in Kemper HCG (ed): Growth, Health and Fitness of Teenagers: Longitudinal Research in International Perspective. Basel, Karger, 1985, pp 81–87.

75   Kemper HCG, Verschuur R: Body build and body composition; in Kemper HCG (ed): Growth, Health and Fitness of Teenagers: Longitudinal Research in International Perspective. Basel, Karger, 1985, pp 88–95.

76   Kemper HCG, Verschuur R: Influence of age, body height and body mass upon physical fitness test results of 12–18 year old boys and girls; in Eiben OG (ed): Current Development in Kinanthropometry. Hum Biol Budapest 1991;18:117–122.

77   Kemper HCG, Verschuur R: Longitudinal study of coronary risk factors during adolescence and young adulthood: The Amsterdam Growth and Health Study. Pediatr Exerc Sci 1990;1:359–371.

78   Kemper HCG, Verschuur R: Longitudinal study of maximal aerobic power in teenagers. Ann Hum Biol 1987;14:435–444.

79   Kemper HCG, Verschuur R: Maximal aerobic power; in Kemper HCG (ed): Growth, Health and Fitness of Teenagers: Longitudinal Research in International Perspective. Basel, Karger, 1985, pp 107–126.

80   Kemper HCG, Verschuur R: Maximal aerobic power in 13- and 14-year-old teenagers in relation to biologic age. Int J Sports Med 1981;2:97–100.

81   Kemper HCG, Verschuur R: Measurement of VO_2max in teenagers with a treadmill test; in Mellerowicz M, Franz I-W (eds): Standardisierung, Kalibrierung und Methodik in der Ergometrie. Erlangen, Perimed Fachbuch-Verlagsgesellschaft mbH, 1983, pp 241–245.

82   Kemper HCG, Verschuur R: Motor performance fitness test; in Kemper HCG (ed): Growth, Health and Fitness of Teenagers: Longitudinal Research in International Perspective. Basel, Karger, 1985, pp 96–106.

83   Kemper HCG, Verschuur R: Other functions; in Kemper HCG (ed): Growth, Health and Fitness of Teenagers: Longitudinal Research in International Perspective. Basel, Karger, 1985, pp 127–136.

84   Kemper HCG, Verschuur R: Physical measurements; in Kemper HCG (ed): Growth, Health and Fitness of Teenagers: Longitudinal Research in International Perspective. Basel, Karger, 1985, pp 35–46.

85   Kemper HCG, Verschuur R, de Mey L, Storm-van Essen L: Longitudinal changes in physical fitness of males and females from age 12 to 23: The Amsterdam Growth and Health Study. Leuven, Hermes, 1990, vol 2–3, pp 299–314.

86   Kemper HCG, Verschuur R, Ritmeester JW: Longitudinal development of growth and fitness in early and late maturing teenagers. Pediatrician 1987;14:219–225.

87   Kemper HCG, Verschuur R, Ritmeester JW: Maximal aerobic power in early and late maturing teenagers; in Rutenfranz J, Mocellin R, Klimt F (eds): Proceedings of the International Symposium of Pediatric Work Physiology. Children and Exercise XII; Hardenhausen, Germany. Champaign, Human Kinetics, 1986, pp 213–225.

88   Kemper HCG, Verschuur R, Storm-van Essen L, van Aalst R: Longitudinal study of maximal aerobic power in boys and girls from 12 to 23 years of age; in Rutenfranz J, Mocellin R, Klimt F (eds): Proceedings of the International Symposium of Pediatric Work Physiology. Children and Exercise XII; Hardenhausen, Grmany. Champaign, Human Kinetics, 1986, pp 203–211.

89   Kemper HCG, Welten DC, Twisk JWR: Weight-bearing activity during youth is a more important factor for peak bone mass than calcium intake (letter). J Bone Miner Res 1995;10:172–173.

90   Kemper HCG, Welten DC, van Mechelen W: Effects of weight bearing physical activity on the development of peak bone density; in Kemper HCG (ed): The Amsterdam Growth Study: A Longitudinal Analyses of Health, Fitness and Lifestyle. Champaign, Human Kinetics, 1995, pp 225–235.

91   Kemper HCG, Welten DC, van Mechelen W, Post GB, Twisk JWR: The role of weight bearing exercise on lumbar bone mass in 27 year old males and females (abstract). Bone 1996;18: 113S–114S.

92   Kemper HCG, Welten DC, van Mechelen W, Twisk JWR: Effects of nutrition and exercise on the peak bone mineral mass of 27 years old males and females (abstract). Sportorvosi Szemle (Hungarian Review of Sports Medicine) 1995;36:51.

93   Kemper HCG (ed): The Amsterdam Growth Study: A Longitudinal Analysis of Health, Fitness and Lifestyle. Champaign, Human Kinetics, 1995.

94   Kilkens OJE, Gijtenbeek BAJ, Twisk JWR, van Mechelen W, Kemper HCG: Clustering of life-style CVD risk factors and its relationship with biological CVD risk factors. Pediatr Exerc Sci 1999;11:169–177.

95   Koppes LLJ: Alcohol Consumption: Results from the Amsterdam Growth and Health Longitudinal Study, Diss. Vrije Universiteit, GIB publ. No. 10, Amsterdam, 2002.

96   Koppes LLJ, Kemper HCG, Post GB, Snel J, Twisk JWR: Development and stability of alcohol consumption from adolescence into adulthood: The Amsterdam Growth and Health Longitudinal Study. Eur Addict Res 2000;6:183–168.

97   Koppes LLJ, Twisk JWR, Snel J, de Vente W, Kemper HCG: Personality characteristics and alcohol consumption: Longitudinal analyses in men and women followed from ages 13 to 32. J Stud Alcohol 2001;62:494–500.

98   Koppes LLJ, Twisk JWR, Snel J, Kemper HCG: Concurrent validity of alcohol consumption measurement in a 'healthy' population: Quantity-frequency questionnaire v. dietary history interview. Br J Nutr 2002;88:427–434.

99   Koppes LLJ, Twisk JWR, Snel J, van Mechelen W, Kemper HCG: Blood cholesterol levels of 32-year-old alcohol consumers are better than of nonconsumers. Pharmacol Biochem Behav 2000;66:163–167.

100 Minck MR, Ruiter LM, van Mechelen W, Kemper HCG, Twisk JWR: Physical fitness, body fatness, and physical activity: The Amsterdam Growth and Health Study. Am J Hum Biol 2000; 12:593–599.

101 Post GB: Nutrition in Adolescence: A Longitudinal Study in Dietary Patterns from Teenager to Adult. Diss, De Vrieseborch/Haarlem, Landbouwuniversiteit Wageningen, 1989.

102 Post GB, de Vente W, Kemper HCG, Twisk JWR: Longitudinal trends in and tracking of energy and nutrient intake over 20 years in a Dutch cohort of men and women between 13 and 33 years of age: The Amsterdam Growth and Health Longitudinal Study. Br J Nutr 2001;85:375–385.

103 Post GB, Kemper HCG: Eating and smoking habits; in Kemper HCG (ed): Growth, Health and Fitness of Teenagers: Longitudinal Research in International Perspective. Basel, Karger, 1985, pp 53–55.

104 Post GB, Kemper HCG: Energy and nutrient intakes, eating and smoking practices; in Kemper HCG (ed): Growth, Health and Fitness of Teenagers: Longitudinal Research in International Perspective. Basel, Karger, 1985, pp 156–168.

105 Post GB, Kemper HCG: Nutrient intake and biological maturation during adolescence. The Amsterdam Growth and Health Longitudinal Study. Eur J Clin Nutr 1993;47:400–408.

106 Post GB, Kemper HCG: Procedures and subjects used in the longitudinal study; in Kemper HCG (ed): The Amsterdam Growth Study: A Longitudinal Analyses of Health, Fitness and Lifestyle. Champaign, Human Kinetics, 1995, pp 6–16.

107 Post GB, Kemper HCG, Storm-Van Essen L: Longitudinal changes in nutritional habits of teenagers: Differences in intake between schooldays and weekend days. Br J Nutr 1987;57: 161–176.

108 Post GB, Kemper HCG, Storm-van Essen L: Snacking habits in Dutch adolescents. Int J Eating Disord 1986;5:85–100.

109 Post GB, Kemper HCG, Twisk JWR, van Mechelen W: The association between dietary patterns and cardio vascular disease risk indicators in healthy youngsters: Results covering fifteen years of longitudinal development. Eur J Clin Nutr 1997;51:387–393.

110 Post GB, Kemper HCG, Twisk JWR, van Mechelen W: Biologic maturation in relation to lifestyle from adolescence into adulthood; in Armstrong N, Kirby B, Welsman J (eds): Proceedings of the International Symposium of Pediatric Work Physiology. Children and Exercise XIX; Exeter (UK). London, E&FN Spon, 1997, pp 53–57.

111 Post GB, Storm-van Essen L, van Aalst R, Kemper HCG: In Hardoff D, Chigier E (eds): Longitudinal Changes in Adolescents and Young Adults. London, Freund Publishing House, 1988, pp 471–485.

112 Post GB, van Zundert A, Kemper HCG: In Frenkl R, Szmodis I (eds): Nutrition in Adolescence and Its Relationship with Biological Maturation. Budapest, National Institute of Health Promotion (NEVI), 1991, pp 157–169.

113 Post GB, Welten DC: The development of nutritional intake during 15 years of follow-up; in Kemper HCG (ed): The Amsterdam Growth Study: A Longitudinal Analyses of Health, Fitness and Lifestyle. Champaign, Human Kinetics, 1995, pp 108–135.

114 Ritmeester JW, Kemper HCG, Verschuur R: Is a levelling-off criterium in oxygen uptake a prerequisite for a maximal performance in teenagers?; in Binkhorst RA, Kemper HCG, Saris WH (eds): Proceedings of the XIth International Symposium of Pediatric Work Physiology. Children and Exercise XI; Papendal, The Netherlands. Champaign, Human Kinetics, 1985, pp 161–170.

115 Schouten WJ, Verschuur R, Kemper HCG: Habitual physical activity, strenuous exercise, and salivary immunoglobulin A levels in young adults: The Amsterdam Growth and Health Study. Int J Sports Med 1988;9:289–293.

116 Schouten WJ, Verschuur R, Kemper HCG: Physical activity and upper respiratory tract infections in a normal population of young men and women: The Amsterdam Growth and Health Study. Int J Sports Med 1988;9:451–455.

117 Snel J, Kempe PT, Kemper HCG: Coronary-prone behavior pattern (type A), personality and health in young men and women; in Coudert J, van Praagh E (eds): Proceedings of the XVIth International Congress on Pediatric Work Physiology. Children and Exercise XVI; St Sauves, France. Paris, Masson, 1992, pp 97–99.

118 Snel J, Kempe PT, van Mechelen W: Longitudinal development of personality; in Kemper HCG (ed): The Amsterdam Growth Study: A Longitudinal Analyses of Health, Fitness and Lifestyle. Champaign, Human Kinetics, 1995, pp 86–106.

119 Snel J, Ritmeester JW: Sociometric status; in Kemper HCG (ed): Growth, Health and Fitness of Teenagers: Longitudinal Research in International Perspective. Basel, Karger, 1985, pp 148–155.

120 Snel J, Twisk JWR, van Mechelen W, Kemper HCG: Effects of adult health of physical condition and lifestyle measured from adolescence through adulthood; in Kemper HCG (ed): The Amsterdam Growth Study: A Longitudinal Analyses of Health, Fitness and Lifestyle. Champaign, Human Kinetics, 1995, pp 247–270.

121 Snel J, van Mechelen W: Lifestyle and health from young adulthood to adulthood; in Kemper HCG (ed): The Amsterdam Growth Study: A Longitudinal Analyses of Health, Fitness and Lifestyle. Champaign, Human Kinetics, 1995, pp 259–172.

122 Storm-van Essen L, Kemper HCG, Ootjers MG: Purpose and design; in Kemper HCG (ed): Growth, Health and Fitness of Teenagers: Longitudinal Research in International Perspective. Basel, Karger, 1985, pp 12–25.

123 Tanashi Satake, Kemper HCG: The Amsterdam Growth Study 20 years-old and the symposium problems and solutions in research. J Hlth Phys Educ Recreation Jpn 1997;13:293–300.

124 te Velde SJ, Twisk JWR, van Mechelen W, Kemper HCG: Birth weight, adult body composition, and subcutaneous fat distribution. Obes Res 2003;11:202–208.

125 te Velde SJ, Ferreira I, Twisk JWR, van Mechelen W, Kemper HCG: Birth weight and musculoskeletal health in adulthood: Result from the Amsterdam Growth and Health Longitudinal Study, 2003, in press.

126 te Velde SJ, Twisk JWR, van Mechelen W, Kemper HCG: Birth weight and musculoskeletal health in adulthood: Results from the Amsterdam Growth and Health Longitudinal Study, 2003, Osteop Int, in press.

127 Twisk JWR: The Design of the Amsterdam Growth and Health Study; in Kemper HCG (ed): The Amsterdam Growth Study: A Longitudinal Analysis of Health, Fitness and Lifestyle. Champaign, Human Kinetics, 1995, pp 6–16.

128 Twisk JWR: Different statistical models to analyze epidemiological observational longitudinal data: An example from the Amsterdam Growth and Health Study. Int J Sports Med 1997;18: S216–S224.

129 Twisk JWR: Tracking of blood cholesterol over a 15 year period and its relation to other risk factors for coronary heart disease, a new methodological approach with data from the Amsterdam Growth and Health Study; Diss. GIB publ. No. 6 Vrije Universiteit, Amsterdam, 1995.

130 Twisk JWR: Physical activity guidelines for children and adolescents: A critical review. Sports Med 2001;31:617–627.

131 Twisk JWR: Physical activity, physical fitness and cardiovascular health; in Armstrong N, van Mechelen W (eds): Oxford Textbook of Paediatric Exercise Science in Medicine. Oxford, Oxford Medical Publications, 2000, pp 253–263.

132 Twisk JWR: Tracking of Blood Cholesterol over a 15 year period and its relation to other risk factors for coronary heart disease: A new methodological approach with data from the Amsterdam Growth and Health Study. Int J Sports Med 1995;18:S216–S224.

133 Twisk JWR, Kemper HCG, Mellenbergh GJ: Longitudinal development of lipoprotein levels in males and females aged 12–28 years: The Amsterdam Growth and Health Study. Int J Epidemiol 1995;24:69–77.

134 Twisk JWR, Kemper HCG, Mellenbergh GJ: Mathematical and analytical aspects of tracking. Epidemiol Rev 1994;16:165–183.

135 Twisk JWR, Kemper HCG, Mellenbergh GJ, van Mechelen W: Factors influencing tracking of cholesterol and high-density lipoprotein: The Amsterdam Growth and Health Study. Prev Med 1996;25:355–364.

136 Twisk JWR, Kemper HCG, Mellenbergh GJ, van Mechelen W: A new approach to tracking of subjects at risk for hypercholesteremia over a period of 15 years: The Amsterdam Growth and Health Study. Eur J Epidemiol 1997;13:293–300.

137 Twisk JWR, Kemper HCG, Mellenbergh GJ, van Mechelen W: Relation between the longitudinal development of lipoprotein levels and biological parameters during adolescence and young adulthood in Amsterdam, The Netherlands. J Epidemiol Community Health 1996;50: 505–511.

138 Twisk JWR, Kemper HCG, Mellenbergh GJ, van Mechelen W, Post GB: Relation between the longitudinal development of lipoprotein levels and lifestyle parameters during adolescence and young adulthood. Ann Epidemiol 1996;6:246–256.

139 Twisk JWR, Kemper HCG, Snel J: Tracking of cardiovascular risk factors in relation to lifestyle; in Kemper HCG (ed): The Amsterdam Growth Study: A Longitudinal Analyses of Health, Fitness and Lifestyle. Champaign, Human Kinetics, 1995, pp 203–225.

140 Twisk JWR, Kemper HCG, van Mechelen W: Prediction of cardiovascular disease risk factors later in life by physical activity and physical fitness in youth: Introduction. Int J Sports Med 2002; 23:5–7.

141 Twisk JWR, Kemper HCG, van Mechelen W: Prediction of cardiovascular disease risk factors later in life by physical activity and physical fitness in youth: General comments and conclusions. Int J Sports Med 2002;23:44–50.

142 Twisk JWR, Kemper HCG, van Mechelen W: The relationship between physical fitness and physical activity during adolescence and cardiovascular disease risk factors at adult age. The Amsterdam Growth and Health Longitudinal Study. Int J Sports Med 2002;23:8–14.

143 Twisk JWR, Kemper HCG, van Mechelen W: Tracking of activity and fitness and the relationship with cardiovascular disease risk factors. Med Sci Sports Exerc 2000;32:1455–1461.

144 Twisk JWR, Kemper HCG, van Mechelen W, Post GB: Clustering of risk factors for coronary heart disease: The longitudinal relationship with lifestyle. Ann Epidemiol 2001;11:157–165.

145 Twisk JWR, Kemper HCG, van Mechelen W, Post GB: Tracking of risk factors for coronary heart disease over a 14-year period: A comparison between lifestyle and biologic risk factors with data from the Amsterdam Growth and Health Study. Am J Epidemiol 1997;145:888–898.

146 Twisk JWR, Kemper HCG, van Mechelen W, Post GB: Which lifestyle parameters discriminate high- from low-risk participants for coronary heart disease risk factors: Longitudinal analysis covering adolescence and young adulthood. J Cardiovasc Risk 1997;4:393–400.

147 Twisk JWR, Kemper HCG, van Mechelen W, Post GB, van Lenthe FJ: Body fatness: Longitudinal relationship of body mass index and the sum of skinfolds with other risk factors for coronary heart disease. Int J Obes Relat Metab Disord 1998;22:915–922.

148 Twisk JWR, Kemper HCG, van Mechelen W, Snel J, Post GB, van Lenthe FJ: Experienced health: Longitudinal relationships with lifestyle and objective health parameters; in Armstrong N, Kirby B, Welsman J (eds): Proceedings of the International Symposium of Pediatric Work Physiology. Children and Exercise XIX; Exeter (UK). London, E&FN Spon, 1997, pp 42–46.

149 Twisk JWR, Snel J, de Vente W, Kemper HCG, van Mechelen W: Positive and negative life events: The relationship with coronary heart disease risk factors in young adults. J Psychosom Res 2000; 49:35–42.

150 Twisk JWR, Snel J, Kemper HCG, van Mechelen W: Changes in daily hassles and life events and the relationship with coronary heart disease risk factors: A 2-year longitudinal study in 27–29-year-old males and females. J Psychosom Res 1999;46:229–240.

151 Twisk JWR, Snel J, Kemper HCG, van Mechelen W: Relation between the longitudinal development of personality characteristics and biological and lifestyle risk factors for coronary heart disease. Psychosom Med 1998;60:372–377.

152 Twisk JWR, Staal BJ, Brinkman MN, Kemper HCG, van Mechelen W: Tracking of lung function parameters and the longitudinal relationship with lifestyle. Eur Respir J 1998;12:627–634.

153 Twisk JWR, van Lenthe FJ, Kemper HCG, van Mechelen W: The longitudinal development of smoking behavior in men and women between 13 and 27 years and the relationship with biological risk factors for cardiovascular diseases. Ned Tijdschr Geneeskd 1995;139:1790–1793.

154 Twisk JWR, van Mechelen W, Kemper HCG, Post GB: The relation between 'long-term exposure' to lifestyle during youth and young adulthood and risk factors for cardiovascular disease at adult age. J Adolesc Health 1997;20:309–319.

155 van Lenthe FJ: The Development of a Central pattern of Body Fat from Adolescence into Adulthood; The Amsterdam Growth and Health Longitudinal Study. Diss, Amsterdam, GIB publ. No. 8, Vrije Universiteit, 1997.

156 van Lenthe FJ, Kemper HCG, Twisk JWR: Tracking of blood-pressure in children and youth. Am J Hum Biol 1994;6:389–399.

157 van Lenthe FJ, Kemper HCG, van Mechelen W: Rapid maturation in adolescence results in greater obesity in adulthood: The Amsterdam Growth and Health Study. Am J Clin Nutr 1996; 64:18–24.

158 van Lenthe FJ, Kemper HCG, van Mechelen W: Skeletal maturation in adolescence: A comparison between the Tanner-Whitehouse II and the Fels method. Eur J Pediatr 1998;157: 798–801.

159 van Lenthe FJ, Kemper HCG, van Mechelen W, Post GB, Twisk JWR, Welten DC, Snel J: Biological maturation and the distribution of subcutaneous fat from adolescence into adulthood: The Amsterdam Growth and Health Study. Int J Obes Relat Metab Disord 1996;20:121–129.

160 van Lenthe FJ, Kemper HCG, van Mechelen W, Twisk JWR: Development and tracking of central patterns of subcutaneous fat in adolescence and adulthood: The Amsterdam Growth and Health Study. Int J Epidemiol 1996;25:1162–1171.

161 van Lenthe FJ, Kemper HCG, van Mechelen W, Twisk JWR: The longitudinal association between physical fitness and fat distribution; in Armstrong N, Kirby B, Welsman J (eds): Proceedings of the International Symposium of Pediatric Work Physiology. Children and Exercise XIX; Exeter (UK). London, E&FN Spon, 1997, pp 57–62.

162 van Lenthe FJ, Snel J, Twisk JWR, van Mechelen W, Kemper HCG: Coping, personality and the development of a central pattern of body fat from youth into young adulthood: The Amsterdam Growth and Health Study. Int J Obes Relat Metab Disord 1998;22:861–868.

163 van Lenthe FJ, van Mechelen W, Kemper HCG, Post GB: Behavioral variables and development of a central pattern of body fat from adolescence into adulthood in normal-weight whites: The Amsterdam Growth and Health Study. Am J Clin Nutr 1998;67:846–852.

164 van Lenthe FJ, van Mechelen W, Kemper HCG, Twisk JWR: Association of a central pattern of body fat with blood pressure and lipoproteins from adolescence into adulthood. The Amsterdam Growth and Health Study. Am J Epidemiol 1998;147:686–693.

165 van Mechelen W, Kemper HCG: Habitual physical activity in longitudinal perspective; in Kemper HCG (ed): The Amsterdam Growth Study: A Longitudinal Analyses of Health, Fitness and Lifestyle. Champaign, Human Kinetics, 1995, pp 135–158.

166 van Mechelen W, Kemper HCG, Twisk JWR, Snel J: Are physical fitness and physiological and psychosocial indices related to sports injuries?; in Kemper HCG (ed): The Amsterdam Growth Study: A Longitudinal Analyses of Health, Fitness and Lifestyle. Champaign, Human Kinetics, 1995, pp 189–202.

167 van Mechelen W, Kemper HCG, Twisk JWR, van Lenthe FJ, Post GB: Longitudinal relationships between between resting heart rate, maximal oxygen uptake and activity; in Armstrong N, Kirby B, Welsman J (eds): Proceedings of the International Symposium of Pediatric Work Physiology. Children and Exercise XIX; Exeter (UK). London, E&FN Spon, 1997, pp 47–52.

168 van Mechelen W, Mellenbergh GJ: Problems and solutions in longitudinal research: From theory to practice. Int J Sports Med 1997;18:S238–S245.

169 van Mechelen W, Twisk JWR, Kemper HCG, Snel J, Post GB: Longitudinal relationships between lifestyle and cardiovascular and bone health status indicators in males and females between 13 and 27 years of age: A review of findings from the Amsterdam Growth and Health Longitudinal Study. Publ Hlth Nutr 1999;2:419–427.

170 van Mechelen W, Twisk JWR, Molendijk A, Blom B, Snel J, Kemper HCG: Subject-related risk factors for sports injuries: A 1-year prospective study in young adults. Med Sci Sports Exerc 1996; 28:1171–1179.

171 van Mechelen W, Twisk JWR, Post GB, Snel J, Kemper HCG: Physical activity of young people: The Amsterdam Longitudinal Growth and Health Study. Med Sci Sports Exerc 2000;32: 1610–1616.

172 van Mechelen W, Twisk JWR, van Lenthe FJ, Post GB, Snel J, Kemper HCG: Longitudinal relationships between resting heart rate and biological risk factors for cardiovascular disease: The Amsterdam Growth and Health Study. J Sports Sci 1998;16:S17–S23.

173 Verschuur R: Daily Physical Activity and Health, Longitudinal Changes during the Teenage Period. Diss, De Vrieseborch/Haarlem, University of Amsterdam and Vrije Universiteit Amsterdam, 1987.

174 Verschuur R, Kemper HCG: Habitual physical activity; in Kemper HCG (ed): Growth, Health and Fitness of Teenagers: Longitudinal Research in International Perspective. Basel, Karger, 1985, pp 56–65.

175 Verschuur R, Kemper HCG: Habitual physical activity in Dutch teenagers measured by heart rate; in Binkhorst RA, Kemper HCG, Saris WH (eds): Proceedings of the XIth International Symposium of Pediatric Work Physiology. Children and Exercise XI; Papendal, The Netherlands. Champaign, Human Kinetics, 1985, pp 194–203.

176 Verschuur R, Kemper HCG: Pattern of daily physical activity; in Kemper HCG (ed): Growth, Health and Fitness of Teenagers: Longitudinal Research in International Perspective. Basel, Karger, 1985, pp 169–186.

177 Verschuur R, Kemper HCG, Besseling CWM: Habitual physical activity and health in 13 and 14 year-old teenagers; in Ilmarinen J, Välimäki I (eds): Proceedings of the International Symposium of Pediatric Work Physiology. Children and Exercise X; Joutsa, Finland. Berlin, Springer, 1984, pp 355–361.

178 Verschuur R, Kemper HCG, de Mey L, Storm-van Essen L, van Aalst R, van Zundert A: Longitudinal development of physical fitness in girls and boys from age 12–22. The Amsterdam Growth and Health Study; in Ruskin H, Simkin A (eds): Physical Fitness and the Ages of Man. Jerusalem, Academon Press, The Hebrew University, 1987, pp 33–58.

Appendix

179   Verschuur R, van Zundert A, Kemper HCG: Longitudinal participation in sports in girls and boys in relation to physical fitness in their late teens and early twenties: The Amsterdam Growth and Health Study; in Ruskin H, Simkin A (eds): Physical Fitness and the Ages of Man. Jerusalem, Academon Press, The Hebrew University, 1987, pp 59–82.
180   Welten DC: Calcium Intake in Relation to Bone Health during Youth: Results from the Longitudinal Amsterdam Growth and Health Study. Diss, Amsterdam, GIB publ. No. 7, Vrije Universiteit, 1996.
181   Welten DC, Kemper HCG, Post GB, van Mechelen W, Twisk JWR, Lips P, Teule GJJ: Weight-bearing activity during youth is a more important factor for peak bone mass than calcium intake. J Bone Miner Res 1994;9:1089–1096.
182   Welten DC, Kemper HCG, Post GB, van Staveren WA: Comparison of a quantitative dairy questionnaire with a dietary history in young adults. Int J Epidemiol 1995;24:763–770.
183   Welten DC, Kemper HCG, Post GB, van Staveren WA: A meta-analysis of the effect of calcium intake on bone mass in young and middle aged females and males. J Nutr 1995;125:2802–2813.
184   Welten DC, Kemper HCG, Post GB, van Staveren WA: Relative validity of 16-year recall of calcium intake by a dairy questionnaire in young Dutch adults. J Nutr 1996;126:2843–2850.
185   Welten DC, Kemper HCG, Post GB, van Staveren WA, Twisk JWR: Longitudinal development and tracking of calcium and dairy intake from teenager to adult. Eur J Clin Nutr 1997;51:612–618.
186   Welten DC, Post GB, Kemper HCG: Bone mineral density and dietary calcium intake; in Kemper HCG (ed): The Amsterdam Growth Study: A Longitudinal Analysis of Health, Fitness and Lifestyle. Champaign, Human Kinetics, 1995, pp 236–246.

Prof. Dr. Han C.G. Kemper
AGAHLS Research Group, Institute for Research in Extramural Medicine
VU University Medical Center
Van der Boechorststraat 7, NL–1081 BT Amsterdam (The Netherlands)
Tel. +31 20 4448407, Fax +31 20 4446775, E-Mail hcg.kemper.emgo@med.vu.nl

Subject Index